Studies in Emotion and Social Interaction

Paul Ekman
University of California, San Francisco

Klaus R. Scherer
Justus-Liebig-Universität Giessen

General Editors

Body Movement and Speech in Medical Interaction

Studies in Emotion and Social Interaction

This series is jointly published by the Cambridge University Press and the Editions de la Maison des Sciences de l'Homme, as part of the joint publishing agreement established in 1977 between the Fondation de la Maison des Sciences de l'Homme and the Syndics of the Cambridge University Press.

Cette collection est publiée en co-édition par Cambridge University Press et les Editions de la Maison des Sciences de l'Homme. Elle s'intègre dans le programme de co-édition établi en 1977 par la Fondation de la Maison des Sciences de l'Homme et les Syndics de Cambridge University Press.

Body movement and speech in medical interaction

Christian Heath

Illustrated by Katherine Nicholls

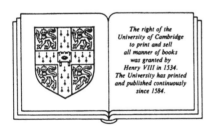

Cambridge University Press

Cambridge
London   New York   New Rochelle
Melbourne   Sydney

Editions de la Maison des Sciences de l'Homme

Paris

CAMBRIDGE UNIVERSITY PRESS
Cambridge, New York, Melbourne, Madrid, Cape Town, Singapore, São Paulo

Cambridge University Press
The Edinburgh Building, Cambridge CB2 2RU, UK

Published in the United States of America by Cambridge University Press, New York

www.cambridge.org
Information on this title: www.cambridge.org/9780521253352

© Cambridge University Press 1986

First published 1986
This digitally printed first paperback version 2006

A catalogue record for this publication is available from the British Library

Library of Congress Cataloguing in Publication data
Heath, Christian, 1952–
Body movement and speech in medical interaction.
1. Physician and patient. 2. Interpersonal
relations. I. Title.
R727.3.H43   1986   610.69′52   85-29998

ISBN-13 978-0-521-25335-2 hardback
ISBN-10 0-521-25335-7 hardback

ISBN-13 978-0-521-03176-9 paperback
ISBN-10 0-521-03176-1 paperback

Contents

Preface

The following book is concerned with some small but not insignificant details of the interaction between human beings. It focuses on the organization of human behaviour in a particular setting, the medical consultation, and explores the coordination between body movement and speech, the visual and vocal aspects of the interaction between the doctor and patient. It is based upon many hours of video recordings of ordinary, everyday general-practice or primary-health-care consultations and involves the detailed analysis of actual examples accompanied by numerous illustrations.

The opportunity to conduct the research which forms the basis of this book derived from my appointment in 1974, on graduating, to the post of Research Fellow in the Department of General Practice, University of Manchester. The head of department at that time, Professor Patrick Byrne, gave his full support and encouragement to the research, and in 1977 we received from the Social Science Research Council research grant HR/5148 to conduct a project concerned with visual and vocal aspects of the general-practice consultation. Following the retirement of Patrick Byrne, Professor David Metcalfe received the chair, and he too provided enthusiasm and support for the research. Without Patrick Byrne, David Metcalfe, and colleagues in the Department of General Practice, especially Alec Brown, Eileen Ineson, Bernard Marks, and Mike Thomas, this research would not have been possible. More recently, I also owe a debt to my colleagues and students at the Department of Sociology, University of Surrey, for providing such a pleasant and stimulating environment for conducting research and teaching related courses. In 1981 the SSRC provided additional support for the research on medical interaction (HR/8143), which provided the opportunity to gather more data and develop and extend the analysis. I should also like to thank Dr. Marshall Marinka and Alan Clarke of the MSD Foundation, London, for making available

a large quantity of excellent-quality video recordings of medical interviews.

Over many years I have been extremely fortunate in receiving detailed
comments and criticism on numerous papers and on presentations at
seminars and conferences; I would like to thank all those who so kindly
showed an interest and helped the research in this way. Max Atkinson,
Charles Goodwin, John Heritage, Gail Jefferson, and Rod Watson deserve
very special mention for their inspiration and support, and for the trouble
they have taken with the analytic concerns and research reported in this
book. I should also like to thank Katherine Nicholls for her artwork and
her patience in producing the many illustrations, and Jackie Little for
her care and perseverance in preparing the manuscript. I am also very
grateful to Sue Allen-Mills of Cambridge University Press for her advice
and general support during the various stages leading to publication
and to Jane Van Tassel for her vigorous copyediting of the final manuscript. Without the delightful companionship of Gillian Nicholls and
the imaginative support of Joan Heath neither the research nor the book
would have been accomplished. It goes without saying that the responsibility for what follows is mine alone.

To all those who so kindly allowed their medical consultations or some
other private exchange to be video recorded in the name of social science,
thank you.

I am very grateful to Routledge and Kegan Paul plc for permission to
use part of an article previously published in *The Sociology of Health and
Illness* (1983.5, 3: 331–4) as the basis to the second part of Chapter 7, and
to reproduce a number of drawings from a different article in the same
journal (1984.6, 3: 311–38) for Fragments 2:6, 2:7, and 2:8. I am also
grateful to Richard Allway of International Distillers and Vintners for
granting permission to use the advertisement for Smirnoff.

C.H.

Market Drayton, Shropshire
1 March 1985

The transcription system

The transcription system for talk was devised by Gail Jefferson and can be found in Atkinson and Heritage 1984; Psathas 1979; and Schenkein 1978; and in more detail in Jefferson 1983a, b, c. The following is an abbreviated version adapted from Jefferson 1983a.

Symbol	*Instance*	*Explanation*
[	Dr: erm: ⌈:: H: ⌊no: ⌈: I haven't W: ⌊well it...	A single left bracket indicates the point at which a current speaker's talk is overlapped by another's talk.
]	Dr: (oh::) ⌈yes⌉ P: ⌊on⌋ my fingers:	A single right bracket indicates the point at which an utterance terminates in overlap with another.
[[	SW: ..getcher::(.)first name J: ⌈⌈Jennifer M: ⌊⌊Jennifer SW: hhhuh hah do: you..	Combined left brackets indicate the simultaneous onset of bracketed utterances.
=	Dr: cheerio= P: =by bye Dr: chee⌈rio Pii ⌊bye	Equal signs, one at the end of a line and one at the beginning, indicate no gap between the two lines.

Symbol		*Instance*	*Explanation*
(0.0)	**Dr:**	**Rob** **(.7)** **Dr: O.kay: Rob**	Numbers in parentheses indicate elapsed time in silence in tenths of a second. In this instance the gap is seven-tenths of a second.
(.)	**F:**	**he got(.)two children..**	A dot in parentheses indicates a tiny gap, probably no more than one-tenth of a second.
_____	**Dr:**	**What's up:?**	Underscoring indicates some form of stress, via pitch and/or amplitude. A shorter underscore indicates a lighter stress than a long underscore.
: :	**Dr:** **P:**	**O:kay?** **(.5)** **so::::**	Colons indicate prolongation of the immediately prior sound. The length of the row of colons indicates the length of the prolongation.
. , ?	**SW:**	**.. feel thats a fair comment? about you**	Punctuation marks are used to indicate intonations, not as grammatical symbols. For example, a question may not necessarily have a rising intonation and so would not receive a question mark.
WORD	**Dr:**	**let me know if there: are any more DIFFICULTIES**	Capitals, except at the beginnings of lines, indicate especially loud sounds relative to the surrounding talk.
< >	**P:**	**..long time actually<I've been about them before**	A greater-than sign indicates a hurried start. A less-than sign indicates a slowing down.

Symbol		Instance	Explanation
º hhh	**Dr:**	**(.6)** **hhhºhh**	A row of *h*'s prefixed by a circle indicates an inbreath; without a circle, an outbreath. The length of the row of *h*'s indicates the length of the in- or outbreath.
º	**P:**	**the:are<ºse se see**	A circle in front of a word or sound indicates that it is uttered at low volume in contrast to the preceding talk. Two circles indicate lower volume still.
( )	**Dr:** **P:**	**its Mister Ho⌈ugh** ⌊**.( )**	Empty parentheses indicate the transcribers' inability to hear what was said. The length of the parenthesized space indicates the length of the untranscribed talk. Parenthesized speaker designation indicates inability to identify a speaker.
(word)	**H:** **P:** **(.4)**	**jus:t the difference** **(yep)**	Parenthesized words are possible hearings or speaker identifications.
(( ))	**Dr:** **(12.00)** **Dr:**	**<so what is it?** **((P. passes bottle))** **I'm not sure I've seen** **these:: before**	Double parentheses contain transcribers' descriptions rather than, or in addition to, transcriptions.

Vocal and visual elements

The following describes the way in which transcripts including both vocal and visual elements are presented in the book. The transcription system used for gaze, details of which can be found below and in C. Goodwin 1981a and Psathas 1978, was devised by Charles Goodwin. It is presented here with a few small modifications.

Transcripts of both vocal and visual elements are normally a small, detailed section of a fragment of talk presented earlier. Unlike transcripts of talk, which are transcribed down the page, one utterance above the other, transcripts including visual elements are transcribed across the page. For example

```
Dr:    What bringesth you this morning
       (.6)
P:     er::m:(.)I've got these::(.)aw:ful spots:
```

is presented in part as

```
P:                  ------er::m:-I've got these::
Dr:    morning
```

So as to capture a spatial representation of the length of silences, gaps are broken down into dashes, each dash equivalent to one-tenth of a second. In this example the "(.6)" gap between the two utterances is transcribed as six dashes.

Relevant visual elements are then mapped onto this transcript with respect to where they occur in relation to the talk and/or gaps. The visual behaviour of the speaker is normally transcribed above the talk, that of the co-participant(s) below. Where, as in a case such as this, we have two speakers, we place one above the other, typically the "main" speaker above, and correspondingly map out the nonvocal elements next to the particular party's talk or line denoted for his or her talk. If details concerning gaze are presented, then the first line or space above or below the talk is reserved for transcribing gaze:

```
                   --------------------'',- _ _ _ _ _ _ _
P:                  ------er::m:-I've got these::
Dr:    morning

                       ···_'',- _ _ _ _ _ _ _
                           ^
                         hand
```

——— The continuous line immediately above or below the transcribed talk and/or silence in this instance indicates that the party is gazing at the face of the co-participant. For a discussion concerning the assessment of gaze direction, in particular towards another, see Chapter 1, especially note 10. In this case the patient is looking at the doctor during "morning" and until the first colon in "er::m:." The doctor gazes briefly at the patient during the "m" sound of "er::m:." If the fragment involves more than two persons, the person being gazed at is indicated on the line.

‑ ‑ ‑ The longer dashes are used to indicate that the party is looking at a particular object; in the case here the doctor and patient turn and look at the patient's hand. Frequently a series of lengthy dashes is accompanied by a description, such as "records," "fingers," "camera," to indicate what object is being looked at.

,,,,,, A series of commas indicates that the party is turning away from a participant. In the example above, the patient turns away from the doctor during "er::m:" and the doctor turns away from the patient towards the end of and following "er::m:."

...... A series of dots indicates that the party is turning towards a co-participant. In the example above, the doctor moves his gaze towards the patient near the beginning of "er::m:." In multiparty interactions, when one party moves his* gaze from one person to another, the notation of dots and commas becomes ambiguous because the person is simultaneously moving away from one co-participant and towards another. On occasions dots and commas are also used to capture gaze moving towards and away from particular objects.

Details concerning the direction of gaze are only presented in transcripts if necessary to the description of a particular fragment. Details of other visual elements are mapped onto the transcript in relation to the talk and gaps, where necessary, in conjunction with gaze or alone. As with gaze, a person's visual behaviour is presented adjacent to his talk or the line reserved for his talk. In the example above it is necessary to present details of a couple of other movements:

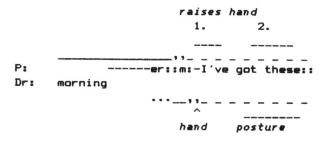

------ Close dashes are used to represent movement. They are accompanied by a description to indicate what type of movement it is. In this instance the patient raises her hand in two moves towards the doctor; the dashes represent the movements. The movement begins initially at the end of "er::m" and ceases near the end of "I've." It restarts at "got" and finishes with "these::." In the area below, we find the doctor moving posturally towards the patient. If necessary, additional dashed lines above and below the transcribed talk are used to represent other movements in relation to where they begin and end in the talk and/or gaps.

*To avoid awkward wording, the masculine pronoun "he" will sometimes be used in the generic sense to mean "he or she."

Some fragments are accompanied by drawings which are based on photographs taken at particular moments. The moments within a fragment from which these pictures are drawn are marked by a "D," typically accompanied by a number to show whether the drawing is the first, second, or *n*th of the action in a particular fragment.

Taking the earlier example we find:

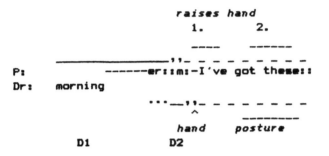

The transcripts that include elements of visual behaviour presented in the book are simplified versions of the more complex maps described in Chapter 1. Coupled with drawings, they are designed to provide the reader with a relatively accessible way of understanding particular aspects of the data. I also provide further details of the particular fragments in the text itself. These ways of presenting a sense of the events are an inadequate substitute for the data itself, the actual videotape recording; they provide the reader with limited access to the precise details with which he might assess the rigour of the arguments and fail to provide the impact and excitement that viewing the phenomena can generate. As discussed in Chapter 1, until we are in a position where actual recordings can accompany text, I hope the method of presentation used here provides an impression of the data without requiring the reader to wade through overcomplicated and turgid detail. One additional difficulty should be mentioned: Even when we are able to accompany text with video recording there may well be some extremely sensitive ethical considerations, and it may be impossible to provide unlimited access to persons' private interactions, especially with the type of data used here. Hence the use of drawings rather than the actual photographs in this book.

1. Video analysis: interactional coordination in movement and speech

If society is conceived as interaction among individuals, the description of the forms of this interaction is the task of the science of society in its strictest and most essential sense.

Simmel 1950, pp. 21–2

This work is part of a program of work undertaken several years ago to explore the possibility of achieving a naturalistic observational discipline that could deal with the details of social action(s) rigorously, empirically, and formally. . . . Our analysis has sought to explicate the ways in which the materials (records of natural conversations) are produced by members in orderly ways that exhibit their orderliness and have their orderliness appreciated and used, and have that appreciation displayed and treated as the basis for subsequent action.

Schegloff and Sacks 1973/1974, pp. 233–4

I want to argue that however rich a researcher's imagination is, if he uses hypotheticalized, typicalized versions of the world, he is constrained by reference to what an audience, an audience of professionals, can accept as reasonable. That might not appear to be a terrible constraint, except when we come to look at the kinds of things that actually occur. Many of the objects we work with would not be accepted as a base for theorizing if they were urged as imagined. We can then come to see that a warrant for using close looking at the world as a base for theorizing about it is that from close looking at the world we can find things that we couldn't, by imagination, assert were there. One wouldn't know they were "typical."

Sacks, quoted in Jefferson 1983b, pp. 17–18

Introduction: medical interaction and video analysis

In recent years there has been a growing interest amongst both medical practitioners and social scientists in communication in the consultation. In the United Kingdom it is especially within general practice or primary health care that we find a growing concern for the relationship and interaction between the doctor and patient. It is now widely recognized

1

that the everyday practice of medicine, the process of diagnosis and prognosis and restoring persons to health and normality, is thoroughly bound up with the ways in which doctors and patients communicate.

Though the significance of communication in general practice had been noted for many years, with discussions on the bedside manner and related subjects, it was perhaps Michael Balint in his classic essay *The Doctor, His Patient and the Illness* (1957) who more than anyone else brought to the profession's attention the importance of communication in the consultation. This is not to suggest that many general practitioners formed or participated in "Balint groups" or were directly influenced by his work. Rather his powerful demonstrations of unexplored illness and the criticalness of communication to diagnosis and treatment permeated the profession and gave support to the growing arguments for postgraduate training and research in general practice.

Amongst the social sciences it is perhaps in sociology that we find the greatest commitment to the analysis of the consultation or, more generally, social interaction in medical settings. As far back as 1935, Henderson, drawing from Pareto, describes physician–patient interaction in terms of the constituent parts of a social system.[1] More important, in 1951 Parsons published his classic *The Social System*, a chapter of which is devoted to an analysis of modern medical practice in relation to the maintenance of social equilibrium, an analysis which provides a rich conception of the mutually compatible roles of physician and patient. This chapter alone not only revealed the significance of doctor–patient interaction to sociological inquiry, but is widely accepted as forming the beginnings of medical sociology itself.[2] However, it was the lectures and essays of Everett Hughes at the University of Chicago in the 1950s which led to the emergence of a wealth of empirical work, largely ethnographic, concerned with social interaction in medical settings.[3] Studies by Becker et al. (1961), Davis (1960, 1963), Glaser and Strauss (1965), Goffman (1961), Roth (1963), Strauss et al. (1964), and many others provide a substantial body of findings and an array of insights concerning the organization of everyday medical practice and the interaction between the profession and its clientele.

Since these studies there has been an immense variety of research conducted on interaction and communication in medical settings. The ethnographic tradition has continued with studies by Emerson (1970), Sudnow (1967), and more recently Strong (1979), and a range of other theoretical and methodological perspectives, both qualitative and quantitative, have been used to examine the behaviour of doctor and patient in the consultation. An important development over the past decade or so has been the use for analysis of audio recordings of actual medical encounters. The recordings provide the researcher with access to detail unavailable to more traditional modes of inquiry such as fieldwork, observation, and interview. The year 1976 saw the publication of the classic *Doctors Talking to Patients,* by Byrne and Long, a detailed study of the verbal behaviours of general practitioners in more than two thousand consultations.[4] Subsequently we have seen the emergence of a range of empirical studies concerned with the details of doctor–patient interaction, especially talk in the consultation, conducted from a variety of perspectives by both social scientists and medical practitioners; see for example the studies reported in Atkinson and Heath 1981; Fisher and Todd 1983; Pendleton and Hasler 1983; and Tanner 1976.

As yet, however, there have been relatively few studies concerned with the visual aspects of behaviour in the medical consultation.[5] One explanation is that it is only recently that a cheap, reliable, and relatively unobtrusive technology for recording vision as well as sound, namely video, has become widely available. More important perhaps is that it is largely psychology and social psychology which have developed empirical research in the area of visual behaviour. The main thrust of this work, but by no means all, is experimental and has necessarily been conducted under laboratory conditions. Consequently studies of naturally occurring behaviour in particular habitats such as the medical consultation are relatively few. An important exception, though it is perhaps inappropriate to consider it in terms of traditional studies of visual communication, is the major body of research which had its beginnings in the work of Bateson, especially Bateson and Mead 1942 and Ruesch and Bateson 1951 and the interdisciplinary collaboration between Bateson, McQuown, Hockett, Birdwhistell, and others in the early 1950s at the Institute of Advanced Study in Palo Alto. The collaborative research at Palo Alto was never published, but it did form the background to Birdwhistell's studies (1970) of body motion and Scheflen's important analysis of psychotherapy sessions (1963, 1966, 1973) and influenced directly and indirectly a range of other empirical work on visual aspects of human behaviour in natural settings, such as Condon and Ogston 1966, 1967, 1971 and Kendon 1967, 1972, 1974a, b, 1977.[6]

In general, sociology, unlike psychology, social psychology, and social anthropology, has been slow to take up the opportunity afforded originally by film and now video.[7] Though there are disadvantages to video in comparison with film, it does provide a cheap and unobtrusive means of recording both the vocal and visual behaviour of human beings *in situ* and subjecting it to close and detailed scrutiny. It provides the facility of making repeated viewings of a fragment of human interaction and the possibility of identifying features of behavioural organization previously unavailable to scientific observation. Moreover video allows the researcher to make available raw data to the scientific community and provide others with the opportunity of evaluating observations and findings, at least in public presentations. On these grounds alone it might be imagined that the emergence of video would have a significant impact on sociology, if not lead to a scientific revolution akin to the impact of the microscope on biology. As yet, however – and we are now into a decade or so of relatively cheap and efficient video technology – sociology has not shown a substantial interest in using the medium for research.

Whatever the financial difficulties of universities both in the United Kingdom and abroad over the past few years, it is unlikely that they explain the near-total absence of video in sociological analysis. The ability to record both the visual and vocal facets of human behaviour may well be irrelevant to certain modes of investigation and sociological concerns; for example, many forms of quantitative analysis might well find no advantage in video technology and the potential it affords. Yet in sociology there is a strong ethnographic tradition, an approach which in various ways emphasizes the importance of grasping the perspectives of the participants and examining social interaction in natural settings. In fact some documentary programmes shown on television are themselves fine examples of ethnography, providing rich insight into the social organization of a particular setting or activity. Sadly, however, ethnographers, save for some important exceptions such as Erickson and Schultz 1982 and Gumperz et al. 1979 which have in general tended to emerge from social anthropology rather than sociology, have fallen behind their colleagues in the media, rarely using video even to supplement the more conventional modes of gathering data. There are of course difficulties of access and recording in some settings of interest to sociologists; more important perhaps is the lack of an analytic framework for handling data collected on video. The theories and concepts conventionally used in ethnography, though finely suited to data generated through fieldwork, observation, and interview, may not, at least as they are traditionally conceived, be applicable to video recordings of actual activities and settings.[8] In examining video recordings of naturally occurring activities, the researcher is faced with a level of detail in human interaction that renders our more familiar sociological concepts and analytic devices somewhat inappropriate save in a very crude sense.

The absence therefore of sociological research using video technology has derived in part from the lack of an analytic framework that can guide the investigation of recordings of naturally occurring actions and activities and their social organization. However, following the major contribution to sociology provided through the work of Harold Garfinkel and in a very different way Erving Goffman, there has emerged in the discipline a form of inquiry that can handle both rigorously and formally the detail provided through audio and video recordings of everyday events; a framework that allows us to explore the social organization of human interaction and the production and coordination of action and activity.[9] Conversation analysis, a development within ethnomethodology, emerged in the 1960s as a result of the pioneering work of the late Harvey Sacks with Gail Jefferson and Emanuel Schegloff. Through their substantial collection of empirical studies, for example Jefferson 1972, 1973, 1974, 1978, 1979, 1980, 1983a, b, c; Sacks 1964–1972, 1972a, 1972b, n.d.; Sacks, Schegloff, and Jefferson 1974; Schegloff 1968, 1972, 1979, 1980, 1984; Schegloff, Jefferson, and Sacks 1977; and Schegloff and Sacks 1973, they have unearthed a hitherto unexplored domain of social organization and provided the methodology and analytic resources to exploit recordings of naturally occurring human behaviour for the purposes of sociological inquiry. Their contribution has given rise to an extensive body of empirical studies concerned with the organization of conversation and the structures of social interaction in a variety of institutional settings. (See for example Atkinson and Drew 1979; Atkinson and Heritage 1984; C. Goodwin 1982; Psathas 1979; Schenkein 1978; *Sociological Inquiry* 1980; *Sociology* 1980; Sudnow 1972; and for a general discussion Heritage 1984a, b and Levinson 1983.)

As the name suggests, conversation analysis has largely been concerned with the social organization of naturally occurring talk, but as video technology has become more widely available a growing number of researchers have begun to investigate the visual as well as the vocal elements of human interaction. As far back as 1964, in his early lectures, Sacks made numerous observations concerning visual behaviour, and in recent years we have seen the emergence of various studies that have used video to explore the social organization of human movement and speech, including Atkinson 1984; C. Goodwin 1979a, 1980, 1981a, 1984, forthcoming; M. H. Goodwin 1980; Goodwin and Goodwin 1982, forthcoming; Heath 1982, 1984a, b; and Schegloff 1984. These studies have begun to reveal a way in which video can be used for the purposes of sociological inquiry and in particular to examine the interactional coordination of social action and activity, whether visual, vocal, or a combination of both.

The chapters collected here are all based upon research that attempts to use video for the purposes of sociological inquiry. The research draws from the methodological resources and substantial body of findings generated in conversation analysis to examine the social organization of certain actions and activities in the medical consultation. In particular the chapters address the moment-by-moment interactional coordination of body movement and speech between doctor and patient. They are based on the detailed analysis of a large collection of video recordings of naturally occurring, everyday medical interactions, predominantly general-practice or primary-health-care consultations. The corpus of data used for the research consists of approximately five hundred hours of video and includes more than a thousand general-practice consultations recorded in a wide variety of practices throughout the United Kingdom. In the course of collecting data over the past decade or so, recordings of other types of interaction, both formal and informal, have been gathered. These include videos of psychiatric and social-work interviews, team and management meetings, receptionists dealing with clients, and conversations in a variety of settings. This relatively large and versatile corpus of data proves very useful during the analysis; it allows one to build large collections of particular phenomena, not infrequently more than two hundred instances of certain action sequences, and compare and contrast a phenomenon across instances, interactions, and settings.[10]

It is hoped that these chapters, in exploring the social organization of movement and speech in the medical consultation, will contribute to our understanding of doctor–patient communication and the growing body of research, in various disciplines, concerned with human interaction. The chapters address various substantive areas within the medical consultation, including the physical examination, leave-taking, and maintenance of involvement, and attempt to cast some light on particular aspects of the interaction between the doctor and the patient. Underlying this interest in the medical consultation is a more general concern with the social organization of movement and speech and the systematics and practical considerations which inform the production and recognition of a range of actions and activities. Consequently it is likely that some of the observations and findings generated in relation to the materials drawn from the consultation hold for social interaction in other settings, both formal and informal. In directing attention towards the medical consultation, I wish to show that though there are features particular to this type of interaction, patients and doctors rely upon and use interactional resources that are not specific to the setting or categories of persons in question. Thus the studies here may be relevant to a range of other work concerned with social interaction not only from within sociology but also in psychology, linguistics, and anthropology. In exploring video recordings of medical interaction it is hoped that the chapters here reveal a little of the organization and structure of the apparent minutiae of social life and capture the delicacy and precision in the articulation of movement and its coordination with speech.

Each of the following chapters is directed towards particular aspects of the social organization of movement and speech in the interaction between doctor and patient. The next chapter rests on examples drawn from the beginning of the consultation and explores the way in which looking at another can serve to initiate action and establish a state of mutual engagement. Chapter 3 develops an issue raised in Chapter 2: the fashion in which talk and in particular an utterance may be coordinated with the visual behaviour of the co-participants. It examines the ways in which speakers may attempt to gain the attention of others through gestures and various forms of body movement and goes on to explore the design of visual behaviour used to maintain a common focus of involvement. These themes inform Chapter 4, where we look at how persons encourage each other to take notice of a particular phenomenon in the local milieu, whether it is a bruised hand or an elaborate gesture. The analysis investigates how people use visual behaviour to fashion the responsibilities and obligations that fellow participants have towards the activity at hand. It attempts to show how involvement in interaction is in a continual state of flux, accomplished moment by moment within the topic or business of the consultation, and reveals the essential contribution that visual behaviour plays in focusing and sustaining our mutual attention.

In exploring the nature of involvement in the consultation, particular interest is given to the ways in which a speaker, be it doctor or patient, can encourage fellow interactants to participate in a certain action or activity. Chapter 5 is rather different. Staying with the themes of involvement and participation, it explores the behaviour of doctor and patient during the physical examination. Far from encouraging each other to heighten their involvement in the business at hand, in the physical examination we find both doctor and patient attempting to disattend to a range of potentially disturbing actions and activities. Temporarily the participants distance themselves from each other and their doings, yet surreptitiously keep an eye on the proceedings and coordinate their visual and vocal action.

Chapter 6 is concerned with the process through which doctor and patient progressively step out of a state of mutual engagement and involvement. It examines the organization of physical leave-taking and shows how it is systematically coordinated with the utterance-by-utterance movement out of the business of the consultation. In the final chapter, a postscript, the opportunity is taken to address some of the more unusual aspects of the interaction between doctor and patient and to discuss the implications of a little of the foregoing to everyday professional conduct. It discusses the use of medical record cards during the consultation and how reading and writing the records can serve to undermine the patients' ability to disclose information and render the doctor insensitive to the moment-by-moment demands of the interaction. The second part of the chapter briefly examines the use of computers during the consultation. It shows how the use of computers generates difficulties not dissimilar to those found with the records, but in addition finds that computers compete for the attention of the doctor and lead to some rather peculiar problems in speaking for both participants.

In a variety of ways therefore the chapters collected here are concerned with two seemingly unrelated themes. On the one hand they address the social organization, the partnership of body movement and speech in the interaction between doctor and patient, and on the other they explore the nature of involvement and the fashioning of participation in the medical consultation. By discussing a range of substantive and analytic issues I hope to demonstrate how the one theme is thoroughly bound up with the other.

The rest of this chapter is concerned with describing a few of the methodological assumptions which underlie this research and its observations.

A methodological note: sequential relations in movement and speech

Conversation analysis rests upon the principle that an utterance can be regarded as an action or activity, produced and recognized in and through a social organization. It has developed the idea, introduced by J. L. Austin (1962) and subsequently elaborated in speech-act theory (cf. Searle 1969), that particular types of utterance, originally referred to by Austin as "performatives," can be said to be doing things with words: "If a person makes an utterance of this sort we should say that he is doing something rather than merely saying something." In numerous empirical studies concerned with the interactional organization of naturally occurring talk, conversation analysis has demonstrated how an immense variety of utterances are found to accomplish social actions and activities and that there is no reason a priori to assume that doing things with words is limited to certain types of utterance. Moreover, in contrast to speech-act theory and other forms of language analysis, it has been cogently shown that an utterance and the action it performs can only be understood with regard to the context in which they occur.

Talk in conversation and throughout a range of formal environments, though by no means all, is organized locally, utterance by utterance, through a systematics which provides for the transition between and allocation of turns at talk one at a time. Within this turn-by-turn, speaker-by-speaker organization, it is found that each next utterance is addressed by its speaker to the local environment of activity and in particular to the immediately preceding action(s), unless, that is, a device is used to display specifically that the utterance is directed to other talk. Speakers design their utterances with regard to prior action(s), and hearers rely upon this local design of actions in order to understand a speaker's particular contribution. Moreover actions are not only designed with reference to preceding actions, but themselves preserve and contribute to the context, advancing the interaction and forming the framework to which subsequent action will be addressed. As Heritage (1984a) has suggested, a current speaker's action is both "context-shaped and context-renewing." Consequently the character of an utterance, an action, or an activity can only be determined, both by participants and analysts, with reference to its location within the local framework of action. As Schegloff and Sacks suggest:

> That is: a pervasively relevant issue (for participants) about utterances in conversation is "why that now," a question whose analysis may also be relevant to find what "that" is. That is to say, some utterances may derive their character as actions entirely from placement considerations. For example, there do not seem to be criteria other than placement (i.e. sequential) ones that will sufficiently discriminate the status of an utterance as a "statement," "assertion," "declarative," "proposition," etc., from its status as an "answer." Finding an utterance to be an "answer," to be accomplishing "answering," cannot be achieved by reference to phonological, syntactic, semantic, or logical features of the utterance itself, but only by consulting its sequential placement, e.g. its placement "after a question." (1973/1974, pp. 241–2)

In addressing the interactional organization of "naturally occurring" talk, conversation analysis has focused upon the organization of structural aspects of social actions and activities. In particular attention has been directed towards the sequential relations which pertain between certain types of utterance and the ways in which actions and activities are conventionally or procedurally accomplished. In general it has been found that almost every action projects a determinate range of possible nexts, providing an opportunity for specific types of subsequent action, and is itself selected from a range of possibilities made relevant by the immediately preceding action(s). The growing body of empirical studies in conversation analysis has identified the sequential relations of a broad range of actions and activities and explored in detail a variety of structural organizations that inform the production and recognition of naturally occurring talk.

Parallel considerations apply to visual behaviour. As with utterances and talk, human movement performs social action and activity. A movement, whether a gesture or postural shift, a nod, or a look, may be used to accomplish particular tasks in face-to-face interaction. Movement performs "locally" and gains its significance through its coordination within the moment-by-moment progression of action or activity, be it vocal, visual, or a combination of both. Moreover there is no reason a priori to assume that doing things visually rather than through speech will be limited to particular types of action or activity, or certain forms of non-vocal behaviour. Rather, as with utterances and talk, it may be fruitful, at least in principle, to consider how the immense variety of movement found in face-to-face interaction may perform social actions and activities. Montaigne captures a flavour of the scope of work accomplished through visual behaviour.

> What of the hands? We require, promise, call, dismiss, threaten, pray, supplicate, deny, refuse, interrogate, admire, number, confess, repent, confound, blush, doubt, instruct, command, incite, encourage, swear, testify, accuse, condemn, absolve, abuse, despise, defy, flatter, applaud, bless, humiliate, mock, reconcile, recommend, exalt, entertain, congratulate, complain, grieve, despair, wonder, exclaim. . . . There is not a motion that does not speak, and in an intelligible language without discipline, and a public language that everyone understands. (1952, pp. 215–16)

As suggested, it has been found that utterances gain their character and interactional significance through their position in a developing stretch of talk and in particular with reference to the immediately prior utterance and utterances. So too with action and activity articulated through movement. For example, whatever the fears that visitors to auctions may suffer, it is extremely unlikely that the odd wave, smile, or wink will be treated by an auctioneer as a candidate bid. For a movement to be treated as a bid, it has to be positioned with respect to the preceding action and the step-by-step progression of the activity. In particular a movement has to be produced in close juxtaposition to an immediately preceding bid or solicit for bids by the auctioneer. The movement gains its local character, its interactional significance, through its location with regard to an immediately prior action and itself forms the basis for subsequent action, perhaps a next bid. Given the enormous variety of physical movements used to produce bids at auctions, we can begin to discern how "placement considerations" are crucial in determining the nature of the action.[11]

In auctions, as in cases where a person may light another's cigarette in response to a request, or pass a particular object, we find examples of the way in which episodes of visual activity may be fitted within and organized in terms of the turn-by-turn structure of talk, the movement gaining the character of a next "turn."[12] Visual action and activity,[13] however, may not necessarily fit within opportunity spaces rendered relevant by an immediately preceding utterance. For example speakers frequently produce nonvocal action and activity alongside an utterance, or a recipient may alter his or her bodily orientation whilst listening to another. Or, as in the following fragment, nonvocal action and activity may be organized almost independently of talk. (The system used to transcribe talk and lay out the visual elements of the fragments of data is described in the front matter of this book.)

Fragment 1:1   Transcript 1

```
        ((Telephone rings))
Dr:     Hello::: (.5) yes dear.. ((Dr engaged on phone))
        (2.3)
A:      °Daddy::
        (.8)
A:      °camera
        (.5)
F:      uh
        (2.2)
A:      kuhhhheh
        (27.00)
Dr:     yues:::.....
```

In this instance the doctor leaves his patient, two young girls and their father, whilst he answers the phone. As the doctor is engaged on the phone, the girls and their father wait in silence save for the few brief vocalizations documented in the transcript. Whilst they wait, the elder of the two girls, Asia, encourages her father to notice the camera, which is lying behind a one-way screen at the side of the surgery.

Fragment 1:1   Transcript 2

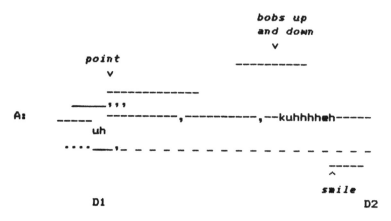

Following the whispered word "camera" the father, who is standing to one side of his seated daughter Asia, begins to turn towards her. As his gaze arrives, Asia throws her head back, raises her eyebrows, and then thrusts her head towards the object in question, the camera.[14] With the head thrust and exaggerated looking, Asia points to the object.[15] As she does, her father turns and looks at the object and Asia produces "kuhhhheh," a sort of laugh smuggled within a cough, and bobs up and down. Continuing to stare at the object, the father smiles. The following drawings, taken at the points marked D1 and D2 in the transcript, will help give a sense of the action.

Fragment 1:1   Drawings 1 and 2

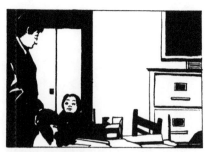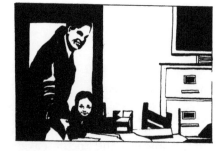

The realignment of gaze by the father, his turning and noticing the camera, is responsive to Asia's head and facial movement, her pointing towards the camera. In pointing, Asia encourages her father to take a look at the camera; her movements generate the relevance of an appropriate next action, an action which should be performed by a particular co-participant in a certain position. Her father's looking at the camera is produced and understood with reference to the preceding movements by Asia and itself provides a basis for subsequent action – the chuckle and mutual appreciation of the object in question. The visual behaviours of Asia and her father lie in immediate juxtaposition, a pair of related actions, where the first encourages the second and the second is responsive to the first.

If we glance back across the fragment, at the participants' behaviour a little before Asia's successful attempt to have her father notice the camera, it also reveals a sense of the sequential relevance of body movement and the ways in which it may render interactional positions for particular types of action and activity. As the girls and their father wait in silence, Asia whispers "°Daddy." Her father turns towards her, and as he does she points to the camera, in a way not dissimilar to the point she provides a second or so later. Her head is thrown back, her eyebrows are raised, and she thrusts towards the object. As she points, her father begins to turn in the direction of the object. The father's movement ceases before his gaze is aligned towards the camera, and Asia, inferring from the movement's completion and the direction of her father's looking that he has not found the object, once again points to the object.

Producing the point provides Asia with the opportunity of inspecting an interactional location in order to discern whether it receives the appropriate response. On producing the action Asia turns to her father and finds that his movements initially fail to accomplish the projected next move. The point provides both the position and the form of action which "should" occur, and its absence is noticeable: A certain type of action generated as relevant in a particular position can be found not to have occurred. In the case at hand, on seeing that her father fails to notice the camera, Asia vocally describes the object in question, whispering the word "°camera." Rather than assisting his search, the whisper encourages the father to turn back to Asia, and as his gaze glides towards her she once again points to the camera, successfully encouraging her father to look at the object in question. Thus the body movement of Asia and her father in Fragment 1:1 begin to reveal how visual action, like vocal, may provide opportunities for subsequent action, encouraging a co-participant to produce a certain type of action or activity in some specific interactional location.

In their classic paper "A Simplest Systematics for Turn Taking in Conversation" Sacks, Schegloff, and Jefferson suggest that the turn organization of talk provides a methodological resource:

> . . . it is a systematic consequence of the turn-taking organization
> of conversation that it obliges its participants to display to each
> other, in a turn's talk, their understanding of other turns' talk. More
> generally, a turn's talk will be heard as directed to a prior turn's
> talk, unless special techniques are used to locate some other talk
> to which it is directed. Regularly, then, a turn's talk will display
> its speaker's understanding of a prior turn's talk, and whatever
> other talk it marks itself as directed to. . . . But while understand-
> ings of other turns' talk are displayed to co-participants, they are
> available as well to professional analysts, who are thereby afforded
> a proof criterion (and a search procedure) for the analysis of what
> a turn's talk is occupied with. Since it is the parties' understandings
> of prior turns' talk that is relevant to their construction of next turns,
> it is their understandings that are wanted for analysis. The display
> of those understandings in the talk in subsequent turns affords a
> resource for the analysis of prior turns, and a proof procedure for
> professional analyses of prior turns, resources intrinsic to the data
> themselves. (1974/1978, pp. 44–5)

Body movement does not necessarily work within the turn-by-turn
structure characteristic of talk, yet the action-by-action character of social
interaction can be used as a resource in analysing movement as well as
speech. As in Fragment 1:1, we can inspect how a visual action or activity
is treated by a co-participant(s) in order to discern his management and
understanding of the preceding and even concurrent movement. Moreover, as studies of conversation demonstrate (cf. Schegloff, Jefferson,
and Sacks 1977), the "third" position in interaction, the action following
the next, is a locus for the initiation of repair. It is a position in which
one party can attempt to initiate repair on, and/or remedy, a difficulty
or misunderstanding displayed in the preceding action and its treatment
of the initial movement or utterance. So for example in Fragment 1:1 we
are able to examine Asia's treatment of her father's response to the original point in order to discern whether it casts any light on her activity.
As we saw, she recycles the action and is successful in encouraging her
father to look at the camera. Thus the progressive step-by-step nature
of interaction provides a methodological resource in analysing the character of actions and activities, be they vocal, visual, or a combination of
both. It provides a way of locating the participants' treatment and understanding of each other's actions and activities, a proof procedure intrinsic to the data.

Body movement also works alongside and within utterances and talk,
yet we can still inspect how particular actions and activities are inter-

actionally managed in order to gain a sense of their character and organization.

Fragment 1:2 Transcript 1

```
P:      Course I've got none now:: li: [ke
Dr:                                    [yeah
        (1.2)
P:      and then when it did strike
        (1.8)
P:      that's it en thats:: sore point about it all::
Dr:     yeah::
P:      when you're never (ea'll) nothing and it does come
Dr:     yeah::< it's all hit you alot of things at once
```

We enter this fragment as the patient is disclosing his difficulties to the doctor. As he produces his utterance "and then when it . . ." he pauses, only continuing the turn following a lengthy (1.8-second) gap. The doctor responds initially with "yeah" and then subsequently with a summary of the impact of the difficulty. Thus the patient's turn "and then when it . . ." is produced and treated sequentially within the talk; it is also coordinated within the course of its articulation with the visual behaviour of the recipient, the doctor.

Fragment 1:2 Transcript 2

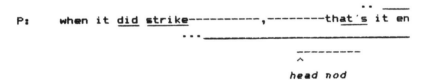

```
P:      when it did strike----------,--------that's it en
```

head nod

The patient withholds the second part of the utterance and roughly 1.5 seconds into the pause[16] the doctor begins to nod. The moment the doctor nods, the patient breaks the pause continuing the turn. The immediate juxtaposition of the head nod and the continuation of the utterance suggests that the first action encourages the second, the head nod perhaps displaying an acknowledgement of or participation in the activity of the patient. The turn at talk itself is the product of interaction between the speaker and the recipient, the doctor's head nod encouraging the production of the utterance.

Moreover speakers themselves engage in movement, gestures, posture shifts, and the like actually within the course of talking, and similarly such movements may be fruitfully investigated with consideration to their interactional organization and the local work they accomplish.

Fragment 1:3   Transcript 1

```
Dr:    you take one of these:: (.4) four times a day
       (.)
P:     yeh
       (.3)
Dr:    erm:: °hh(.)and it(.)often::: (1.5) they help sort
       of (.3) you know dampen down:: any inflamation
       inside the knee (.2) as well(.)alright
       (.)
Dr:    hhh so if you rest for a bit ....
```

We enter towards the end of the consultation as the doctor describes the treatment he is giving and its effects. As the doctor utters "they help sort of (.3) you know dampen down::" he produces a gesture. The gesture illustrates dampening down: The hand is raised with the palm flat and thrust up and down a number of times.

Fragment 1:3   Transcript 2

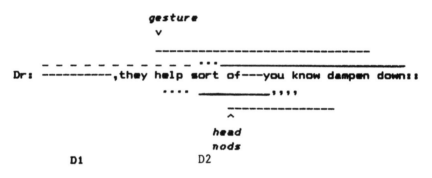

As the doctor begins to describe the effects of the treatment he stops writing and turns towards the patient; the patient is looking down towards the floor. The doctor begins the gesture, and as the hand is raised the patient turns from the floor to the doctor. The doctor continues to gesture, successively moving the hand up and down, and the patient, looking at the doctor, produces a series of head nods in time with the movements of the gesture. More precisely, as the doctor's hand passes down to illustrate dampening, the patient dips his head; as the hand is raised, the head is raised; and so it continues for three "dampenings" in total. The patient's movements are delicately and precisely coordinated with those of the speaker, almost mimicking with the head the illustration articulated with the hand.

Fragment 1:3   Drawings 1 and 2

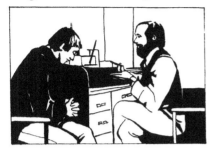 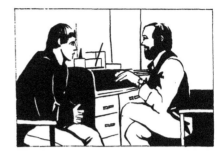

The doctor's gesture appears to illustrate the vocal description it accompanies, elaborating the effects of the treatment and presumably informing the patient's interpretation of the utterance. Vocal and visual are packaged together to accomplish a particular activity. Yet in examining the articulation of the gesture and the behaviour of the co-participant we can begin to discern related interactional work that the movement accomplishes.[17] Whilst illustrating the accompanying talk, the gesture initially serves to encourage the recipient to turn towards the speaker. As the gesture progresses, the recipient begins to respond with a series of head nods coordinated with the speaker's hand. The gesture performs particular actions in the course of its articulation, encouraging the recipient to participate in the activity. It serves to transform the environment in which the activity is received and gains an active and visually orientated recipient. Consequently, in exploring the action(s) a movement accomplishes, it is helpful to examine how it is dealt with both during and following its production and to consider "why this now": How does the person's conduct assist or deal with the circumstances at hand? Certain components of a body movement may implicate action by others whilst forming part of an overall activity accomplished with talk.

In exploring the interactional organization of movements such as the gesture in Fragment 1:3 we can also consider how this brief activity – no more than a second or so in duration – is sensitive to the contingencies at hand and the tasks it is performing. Not any movement the doctor could produce would serve to illustrate the particular effects of the treatment or encourage the co-participant to realign his gaze and nod his head. In different circumstances similar types of action would inevitably have to be produced using very different forms of movement. To perform particular actions within some interactional context, the movement has to be designed, articulated so as to accomplish certain types of work with respect to features of the context at some "here and now." Action and activity through movement are far from idiosyncratic, characterless, or determined; they are accomplished and interactionally coordinated anew on each and every occasion.

Like speech, human movement accomplishes social action and activity, action and activity that rely upon and are articulated through a social organization, a publicly available collection of procedures that provide for their production and recognition. Movement stands in a variety of relations to speech. Even in the few examples discussed here, it has been seen how movements may stand alone, be coordinated with preceding talk or related to both concurrent vocal activity and surrounding nonvocal actions. Actions and activity performed through movement achieve their character and local impact through their position in the context at hand and in particular with reference to the immediately preceding and frequently concurrent activity, be it vocal or nonvocal. Whilst addressing context, movement contributes to and progresses the context and renews the environment of activity. Human movement in interaction may serve to deal with prior action and implicate subsequent activity; it can work on behalf of concurrent activity or initiate a string of events; it provides options and opportunities for following action and activity and is itself selected from a range of alternatives rendered relevant through preceding action and activity. Action and activity accomplished through movement, speech, or a combination of vocal and visual are sequentially organized. It is this social organization, the procedures and reasoning it entails, which forms the central focus of the following studies, a sociological investigation of body movement and speech in medical interaction.

The local geography of action

The interactional position of an action or activity, be it vocal, nonvocal, or a combination of both, is crucial to the determination of its character, operation, and organization. Repeated viewings alone of video data[18] are inadequate in attempting to locate the precise position of the various elements of a particular fragment. Viewing the actual data – the video recording – needs to be augmented by a way of documenting the local geography of action and the location of the various elements and their interrelation at some point in the data. In the course of the research reported here, a rough-and-ready procedure was developed for mapping fragments of data, a method drawing on other systems of transcribing the data for the purposes of analysis. Like all systems of transcription, the method discussed here is selective (cf. Ochs 1979) and focuses especially on the sequential aspects of the action. It is not, nor could it be, an attempt at literal description: The video recording is the actual data; the process of mapping fragments is simply an analytic device for developing a sense and picture of its detail.

Conversation analysis and ethnomethodology are fortunate in having available a widely used transcription system for talk. The system has been developed over a number of years by Gail Jefferson; it captures the details of speech as it is spoken and focuses in particular on the sequential features of talk. It is described in the front matter of this book. The vocal elements of the data are transcribed using this system and then transferred to graph paper to enable visual elements to be mapped onto the transcript of the talk. In transferring the transcript of the talk to graph paper, the talk of each speaker is laid out across the page rather than vertically turn by turn, each speaker's utterance continuing horizontally where the previous speaker ceased talking, or following the appropriate gap. So as to capture a spatial representation of silences and pauses, a single dash is used to represent one-tenth of a second, so that a 0.7-second gap would be represented by seven dashes. If we take a transcript of a brief fragment of talk as in the first transcript below, we can see in Transcript 2 how a section of it has been laid out across the page.

Fragment 1:4 Transcript 1

```
        (20.00)   ((Dr writes))
Dr:     Ri::ght(.)O.kay::?
        (.2)
P:      Oakay
        (.)
Dr:     Ri:ght(t) fi [ine
P:                    [Thank you very mu [ch
Dr:                                      [O.kay?
        (.3)
Dr:     By [e::
P:         [(--,--,)
        (.3)
P:      By [e
Dr:        [Terra::
P:      Bye
```

Fragment 1:4 Transcript 2

```
Dr:   Ri:ght(t) fi [ine                    [O.kay?---By [e::
P:                 [Thank you very mu [ch               [(---,
```

Some fragments of data may not entail talk. Thus the vocal elements of the data cannot be used as a standard on which to transcribe the visual behaviour. In such cases it may be possible to use a particular activity as a standard to which to relate other visual elements of the data. If not, or perhaps in conjunction, one can draw a standard time scale on the graph paper and lay out the details of visual behaviour in relation to clock time.[19] However, it is found that, even in cases where the data has a split-second time record on the tape, it is far more difficult to locate the various visual elements with respect to a time scale than it is to a detailed transcription of the talk.

A long-standing problem for both students and teachers of human movement has been the absence of a general and widely accepted transcription system. For example in his neoclassical study on the principles of public speaking Gilbert Austin suggests: "One of the reasons which may be assigned for the neglect of cultivating the art of gesture, is the want of copious and simple language for expressing its modifications with brevity and perspicuity" (1806, p. 271). He continues by providing a detailed orthography for representing visual behaviour in relation to oratory and drama. More recently we have seen the emergence, in various disciplines, of systems for transcribing aspects of human movement and expression (see for example Birdwhistell 1970; Bull 1981; Ekman and Friesen 1978; Hall 1963; Laban 1956; Laban and Lawrence 1947; and for a general discussion Kendon 1982a). As Kendon (1982a) suggests, the various systems deal with particular aspects of human movement and expression and are designed to address particular problems and serve certain purposes and modes of investigation. Given the variety of concerns and assumptions found even within research on nonverbal communication, coupled with the fact that no system could claim to be a literal representation of the events, it is extremely unlikely that Austin's hope of a single, widely accepted system for transcribing visual behaviour will emerge. Particular transcription systems are suitable for certain types of research and irrelevant for others; consequently as studies of human movement and expression continue to develop it will continue to be necessary to retain and create a variety of transcription systems.

In conducting the research reported here, a number of transcription systems for visual behaviour were experimented with, including those used in dance (Laban 1956) as well as nonverbal communication (Birdwhistell 1970; Hall 1963). After successive attempts to use various systems, it was decided that it would be more suitable to use a method of mapping out the data; not dissimilar to procedures employed in other

studies of visual and vocal behaviour, especially those found that focus
on the interactional coordination of movement and speech (cf. Condon
and Ogston 1964, 1966, 1967; Kendon 1967, 1974, 1977; and Scheflen
1966, 1973).[20] Within this process of mapping the video data, one transcription system did prove extremely useful. That is the orthography
developed by C. Goodwin (1979a, 1980, 1981a) for capturing gaze, a system designed to work alongside the system created by Jefferson for the
transcription of talk in interaction. Goodwin's system is described in the
front matter of the book. In mapping visual and vocal elements of the
data onto graph paper, the first line above a participant's talk is dedicated
to tracking the details of his gaze.[21]

Fragment 1:4 Transcript 3   (Gaze)

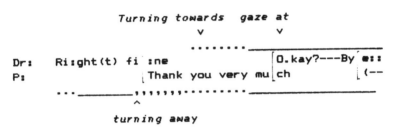

Additional lines of close dashes above the locus for a participant's talk
and the line devoted to tracking gaze are used to capture other aspects
of visual behaviour in which a participant engages. A particular line is
dedicated to tracking the movement of a particular body part, for example
a leg or torso. A line is used to track the behaviour of a particular part
of the body only if movement occurs; so for example if a person's postural
orientation remains stable through a particular fragment it is not tracked
on the graph. A line is used to indicate that a movement is occurring.
Where the line begins marks its point of start; where it ends, its completion. Additionally arrows are sometimes used to indicate the direction
of the movement and particular changes in its character, and greater-
than and less-than signs ($>$, $<$) to capture points of acceleration and de-
celeration. For various purposes an array of other symbols may be used
to elaborate certain details. The following is a section of Fragment 1:4
mapped out as if on graph paper; it captures approximately three seconds
of interaction. It sketches movement in relation to surrounding movement and speech in the closing section of a consultation. The couple of
drawings taken at points D1 and D2 may help to provide an additional
sense of the action.

Fragment 1:4   Transcript 4

```
leg l/h        _____
posture        _____
gesture l/h    _____                                          __
head                                                _____
gaze                                    ........_____
Dr:        Ri:ght(t)  fi ⌈:ne              ⌈O.kay?---By ⌈e::
P:                      ⌊Thank you very mu ⌊ch          ⌊(-
gaze           ...._____,,,,,,,,,,,........_____
head           _____
gesture r/h    _____  _ _ _ _ _  _____
posture        ____                         _____
leg l/h        _____              __
leg r/h                                     _____  __
               D1                                           D2
```

Fragment 1:4   Drawings 1 and 2

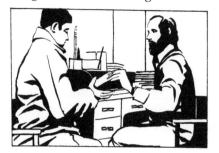 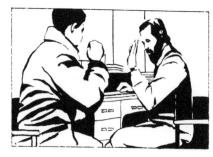

The map and the process of laying out a fragment of data in this way are solely an analytic device, a way of locating a few behavioural details. The map stands as a simplified representation of a few seconds of human interaction, a sketch of the local geography of the movement and speech of all the participants in a particular domain. It is an analytic device for determining the range of human movement within a fragment, frequently allowing the observer to notice phenomena that were missed even after repeated viewings of the data. Moreover the process of mapping not only helps the researcher see behaviour that might otherwise pass unnoticed but allows him to locate the precise position of visual and vocal behaviour within a short stretch of interaction; to sketch out what happens where, what occurs with what, and what precedes and follows particular behaviours within the moment-by-moment coordination of human activity. The map is used in conjunction with the actual data, the video recording, and helps the observer explore the possible relations between the various movements and speech of the participants. From there we can begin to develop an understanding of the local framework of visual and vocal behaviour and attempt to explicate the packaging and structure of action and activity, whether through movement or speech or a combination of both, in a brief fragment of social interaction.

In the research reported here the process of mapping and analysing the video recordings was guided by an interest in particular phenomena. No attempt was made to transcribe all the data in the way described; given the amount of data and the depth of the analysis this would have been impossible. More important, though, the concern of the research was to identify the organization of particular action sequences and the structure of certain activities; this is only possible by comparing and contrasting a large number of instances drawn from a range of consultations; hence much of the data for these particular purposes prove redundant. In developing an interest in a particular phenomenon all the "possible" instances from the whole corpus of data are copied onto a specific tape(s) and then broken down and analysed in detail. As the analysis develops, further searches are made through the whole data corpus for instances that may originally have been missed, or for phenomena now seen as related, and these are then subject to detailed examination. As observations and findings emerge, and different types and variations of particular phenomena are identified, the video-recorded and transcribed collection of instances is reedited in terms of specific themes and categories of phenomena. It is not unusual for a recorded collection to contain two or three hundred instances of a particular phenomenon subdivided into various types. In the course of investigating particular actions and scavenging through the corpus of video recordings to find additional instances, other phenomena are discussed which may have little to do with the concern at the time. These phenomena, again gathered into collections and edited onto particular tapes, are not infrequently studied in their own right at some later date. Thus further phenomena for study continually emerge in the course of detailed analysis.

As mentioned earlier (in the discussion of the transcription system), for the purposes of presenting fragments of data in the book, simplified transcripts, drawn from the more complex maps, are used. In many cases these are accompanied by drawings, taken from the video at particular moments, and chosen to crudely capture a body movement or change in the participants' orientation.[22] Moreover for reasons of space and to make the discussion more readable I have severely limited the number of instances of particular phenomena and the detail in which they are examined in each chapter, only selecting a few of each case so as to capture very briefly both the typicality of and variation in the organization of particular activities. None of this is any substitute for the actual data or more detailed examination; should these be of interest I would be more than pleased to present and discuss the actual video recordings and their analysis.

2. The display of recipiency and the beginning of the consultation

In the external demeanour nothing will be found so effectually
to attract attention, and to detain it, as the direction of the eyes.
It is well known that the eyes can influence persons at a
distance; and that they can select from a multitude a single
individual, and turn their looks on him alone, though many lie
in the same direction. The whole person seems to be in some
measure affected by this influence of another's eyes, but the
eyes themselves feel it with the most lively sensibility.

G. Austin 1806, p. 101

In the beginning of the consultation the participants move from the preliminaries to the business at hand, the reason for the patient's visit.
Greetings are exchanged, identities checked, the patient establishes an
appropriate spatial and physical orientation, and the doctor sorts out
equipment and documentation, not infrequently reading the medical record cards. These preliminaries entail a variety of concerns: a constant
shifting of attention in which the participants are more or less aware of
each other's actions and activities; a fragmentation of involvement, and
necessarily so. In contrast, movement into the business of the consultation establishes a mutual focus of involvement, a stretch of continuous
activity that concerns both participants and requires their coordination
and joint attention.

Looking at one another plays a significant part in the process of establishing a common focus of activity and involvement, not simply as a
means of monitoring each other's concerns and behaviour, but actually
in initiating action and activity. A look can affect another in some way;
it can give rise to a particular impression and encourage others to engage
in certain behaviour – characteristics and consequences of human regard
which have not passed unnoticed in literature and the sciences. Novelists
for example may use a person looking at another to capture influence

and assertion and looking away to reflect shyness, modesty, and even guilt. In the sciences, for example ethology, it has been found that threat displays may be initiated through looking (cf. Hall and Devore 1965; Hinde and Rowell 1962) and it has been shown how certain species undergo a marked shift in electrical activity when looked at (cf. Wada 1961). In the human sciences, the look – or better perhaps gaze – has long been of interest; for example both Simmel (1952, 1969) and Sartre (1956) in very different ways expose the effects of looking at another and the experience which derives from an exchange of glances. And in more recent years there has emerged a substantial body of research concerned with the organization of looking and its influence on others; in particular there has been a growing recognition that looking itself may perform social action and activity and gain its significance through systematic use in face-to-face interaction.[1]

In this chapter I wish to explore the way in which looking, or gaze, is employed to initiate and progress action and activity within the medical consultation. In particular the concern is with the way in which talk may be coordinated with another's gaze and how gaze serves to encourage the production of an utterance. Many of the examples will be drawn from the beginning of consultations, and towards the end of the chapter some remarks will be addressed to how gaze plays a significant part in the achievement of certain formal characteristics of medical interviews.

An initial curiosity in the consequences at looking at another and withholding gaze was raised in coming across the following fragment.

Fragment 2:1 Transcript 1

```
Dr:   Hello
P:    hello
Dr:   come in Missus Lebling
      (3.3)
Dr:   Sit down please
      (9.0)
Dr:   Yes(.)what can I do for you?
P:    Ohhh well(.)since urm (.5) last Friday I've not
      been very well Doctor Jerousa
Dr:   yes
P:    I've been very depressed
Dr:   mmm mhuh
P:    an I feel as though all me inside is breakin up
      (.3)
Dr:   um::
P:    Ohhh I can't eat an I can't sle:ep Ohhh and erm:::
Dr:   for how long have you been like that
```

Like others discussed in this chapter, it is drawn from the beginning of the consultation. It is here that patient and doctor establish co-presence and move from the preliminaries to the business at hand. The patient enters and greetings are exchanged. She then crosses the room, sits down, and assumes a postural and facial orientation towards the doctor as he asks her to sit. There the patient sits in silence until the doctor initiates the business of the consultation with "Yes(.)what can I do for you?" Throughout the silence the doctor reads the medical record. The patient waits, facing the doctor though not looking at him; in fact she sits with her eyes closed, only opening them when he begins to talk.[2]

Fragment 2:1 Drawings 1 and 2

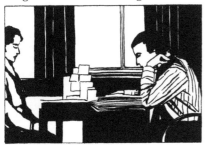 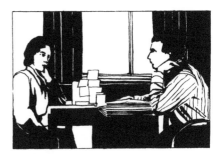

```
         D1                    D2
Dr:    -----------,-----------Yes(.)what can I ...
```

Gaze and the elicitation of talk

In Fragment 2:1 the doctor introduces talk, initiating the business of the consultation as he finishes reading the medical records. In other cases a person who begins to speak following a silence may be encouraged to do so by the co-participant.

Fragment 2:2 Transcript 1

```
Dr:    Hello
P:     Hello
Dr:    Mohammed Oola?
P:     Yes
Dr:    Yes could you sit down(.)please
       (7.3)
Dr:    What can I do for you?
P:     Ohhh (.2) um:: (.7) um::: last week on our:::::fff
       holiday
```

As with the previous example, there is a silence between the request that the patient sit down and the initiation of the business of the consultation by the doctor with "What can I do for you?" The patient begins to sit during the doctor's request, and as he lands moves forward to one side and then back in his chair. Neither the patient nor the doctor looks at the other, the patient looking away from the doctor and the doctor reading the medical records. Remaining still for a second or so, the patient then shifts posturally towards the doctor and simultaneously turns and looks at his cointeractant. Immediately following the patient's movement forward and his gaze shift,[3] the doctor begins to speak, producing the utterance which initiates the business of the consultation.

Drawings 1 and 2

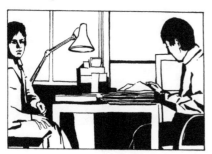 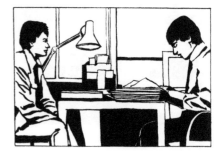

Fragment 2:2 Transcript 2

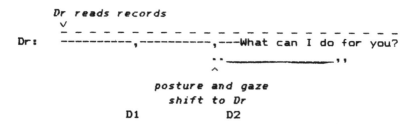

During the silence of seven seconds or so, either party might have spoken, freely choosing from a range of positions to initiate action or activity. The silence is an environment of free-floating opportunity, available for use whenever either party might desire. Within this environment, however, the doctor does not begin to speak as in Fragment 2:1 on finishing an inspection of the records; in fact he continues to read as he speaks to the patient. Rather the doctor's utterance occurs in immediate juxtaposition to the visual actions of the patient, the postural movement and realignment of gaze. It is as if by turning towards the doctor the patient encourages him to speak, the patient's movements breaking the environment of undifferentiated opportunity and marking a position where the other "should" produce an action or activity.

It is useful to refer to the way in which a person may present himself through gaze and sometimes posture towards another as a display of recipiency. Through a display of recipiency an interactant may show that he is ready and prepared to receive an action or activity from another person. The close juxtaposition of the doctor's utterance and the display of recipiency suggests that the first action might in some way elicit the second, the patient gently pushing the doctor into the business of the consultation.

It is worth considering another couple of examples, both again drawn from the beginning of the consultation, in particular the lapse between the preliminaries and the start of business – the discussion of the patient's complaint.

Fragment 2:3   Transcript 1

```
Dr:     Come:in::
        (.3)
        (door opens)
P:      He⌈llo there
Dr:      ⌊hello
        (.7)
Dr:     Mississ Hodgshin
        (.)
P:      yes::
        (2.7)
Dr:     Like to take a seat
        (1.5)
Dr:     Howav:: you bee:n:
```

Fragment 2:3   Transcript 2

```
        Dr reads records
        _ _ _ _ _ _ _ _ _ _ _ _ _ _ _..__
Dr:     -----------,-----Howav:: you bee:n:
                     .._____
        ^
        P sits and aligns posture
```

The patient lands in the chair approximately 0.8 second into the 1.5-second silence. The doctor is reading the records and only brings her

gaze towards the patient at the completion of her initiating utterance.
On landing in the chair the patient moves posturally backwards, progressively bringing her body into an alignment with the doctor. Half a
second or so after landing, the patient turns and looks at the doctor; the
moment her gaze arrives, the doctor breaks the silence and begins to
speak, producing "Howav:: you bee:n:." The utterance appears to be
coordinated with the patient's nonvocal action, the display of recipiency.

The following example is slightly different. The doctor attempts to
initiate the business of the consultation with a two-part utterance separated by a pause. Rather than initiating a disclosure from the patient
concerning "what the problem is" or "how it has been," the utterance
attempts to encourage a review of the previous consultation:

Fragment 2:4   Transcript 1

```
Dr:     Hello
P:      Hello
        (.2)
Dr:     Ohhh (.5) its Mister Kou[gh::
P:                              [(   ) (.) No Hough
Dr:     Yes yes
        (.5)
Dr:     Just come in an:: sit down Mister Hough
        (.7)
Dr:     Er:: (.4) you saw Doctor Lehar::
        (.3)
P:      ah
Dr:     a fortnight ago
P:      two weeks ago
Dr:     two weeks ago
        (1.0)
Dr:     cos you were getting::?
P:      um:: (.3) gastric ulcer
```

Fragment 2:4   Transcript 2

```
        _ _ _ _ _ _ _ _ _ _ _ ··_____
Dr:     Mister Hough-------err::-----you saw Doctor hehar::
                          ··_____
                                         ''
```

The first part of the doctor's utterance "err::" is content-free; it projects
more to follow and transforms the silence into a pause within the utterance of the doctor. The beginning of the "content" of the utterance
"you saw Doctor Lehar::" appears to be coordinated with the doctor
finishing the activity with the records; as he questions the patient he

looks up, ceasing to write. The first part of the utterance "err::" which breaks the silence is juxtaposed with the patient turning towards the doctor; it responds to a display of recipiency. Thus the doctor's utterance is coordinated with his own nonvocal activity and that of his recipient. He responds to the patient's gaze shift with "err::," a content-free component which allows him to take the floor to speak but delays the actual activity until he has finished reading the records. Though not ready to begin, the doctor acknowledges the patient's nonvocal action, the shift of gaze, and produces a response, transforming the environment from one of open opportunity to his responsibility at some particular moment.[4]

In the preceding examples we find the patient and the doctor momentarily disengaged from mutual involvement before moving into the business of the consultation, a mutual activity and a common focus of attention. The patient establishes co-presence and renders himself available, and the doctor reads the medical records. The display of recipiency initiates movement into a state of mutual engagement concerned with the patient's reason for the visit. A state of temporary disengagement and lapses in talk may, however, occur elsewhere in the consultation,[5] and on such occasions a display of recipiency may serve to reestablish talk and mutual involvement. In the following fragment the patient is drawing to a completion the description of her difficulties and appears progressively to disengage from the doctor.

Fragment 2:5 Transcript 1

```
Dr:   ye::r:s:: [:
P:              [an I  jus:t ca:n:t: move:: at all now:
      (.2) and I can't sleep at night: and he gave me
      aspirins to ta:ke a(t) night:
      (.)
P:    Ohhhh
      (.2)
P:    en theyer:: just:t(.)pointless taking them doctor
      (1.0)
P:    Otch
      (.5)
Dr:   Ohhhhhh right(.)well theres quite alot in
      tha::t(.)lets:: jus:t:(.)err:: (1.0) give me a
      moment to recap because I haven't seen you
      before::
```

Coupled with the utterance "en theyer:: just:t . . ." are a number of head nods through which the patient progressively turns away from the doctor. The movements, coupled with the intonation contour of the utterance, a sharp fall towards its close, indicate that the patient is drawing her disclosure to an end and has nothing more to add. Moreover the movements and the utterance provide the impression that the patient is disengaging from the doctor, relinquishing the floor and stepping back from her co-participant. The doctor does not speak, and a silence of one second ensues, with the participants orientated away from each other. The patient breaks the silence with "°tch," a clicking sound made with the tongue, a vocal shrug.[6] The sound reemphasizes that the patient has nothing more to add and puts a little pressure on the doctor to speak. There is no response, and less than half a second later the patient turns and looks at the doctor.

Fragment 2:5   Transcript 2

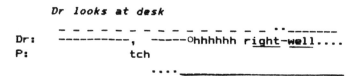

```
        Dr looks at desk

        _ _ _ _ _ _ _ _ _ _ _ _ _ _ _ ··_____
Dr:     ----------,  -----°hhhhhh right-well....
P:                tch
        · · · ·_____
```

The moment the patient looks at the doctor he takes a lengthy inbreath and then begins to speak. As with the previous examples, the vocalization which breaks the silence immediately follows the patient's visual action, a realignment of gaze. The display of recipiency serves to encourage talk following a temporary lapse, and to refocus the involvement of the interactants. But even though the doctor does respond to the patient's nonvocal action and reintroduces talk, it is interesting to observe that he begins with a lengthy inbreath which actually postpones producing an immediate answer to the patient's complaint. Like "err::" in Fragment 2:4, the inbreath simultaneously acknowledges the patient's action but delays the actual reply; it temporarily copes with the sequential implication of the gaze shift but fails to provide immediate assistance for the patient's difficulties. It reveals the way in which turning and looking can place another under pressure to respond even though the co-participant has at that moment nothing more to say.

In Fragment 2:5 as in earlier extracts we find examples of the way in which visual behaviour may serve to encourage another to talk. Simply turning towards another can form the first move out of a temporary lapse in the consultation, one person gently pushing another into initiating an activity. However slight or delicate, the display of recipiency transforms the local environment, carving up the silence and encouraging a co-participant to reengage a state of mutual involvement. Thus the display of recipiency, even if no more than a seemingly minute shift in visual focus, is interactionally significant; it is sequentially implicative, encouraging another to respond at a particular moment and forming the first action of a two-action sequence. The sequential relevance of a display of recipiency places the other under an obligation to produce an action; it marks a moment within the interaction where one party might be expected to respond to the other. Kendon in his classic paper on some functions of gaze direction makes a related point concerning the consequence of being looked at:

> When one perceives another is looking at one, one perceives that the other intends something by one, or expects something of one. In a word, one is being taken account of by another. It seems reasonable to suppose that this will have quite marked arousing consequences, but what line of action it arouses one to take will depend upon the context in which the Look is perceived. (Kendon 1967/ 1977, p. 51)

In an earlier example it was observed that throughout a silence within the beginning of a consultation a patient, though facing the doctor, sat with her eyes closed. Considering the other instances, one can begin to discern some interactional reasons for behaviour which might initially appear rather unusual. Presenting herself both facially and posturally towards the doctor but not looking at him allows the patient to make herself available for interaction.[7] The patient awaits the doctor's pleasure and provides the cointeractant with an open and unconstrained opportunity to initiate action when he so desires.[8] The patient displays a state of readiness, of continued availability, prepared to enter into activity at the instigation of her cointeractant. Closing her eyes allows the patient both to display availability and avoid displaying recipiency; the doctor remains unconstrained and unencouraged to initiate action and activity, at liberty to start when he so wishes.

The display of availability and the display of recipiency are two very different types of action. The display of availability is an action that creates, for its recipient, a range of undifferentiated opportunity in which to initiate action. It is a preinitiating activity, allowing an actor to proclaim that he is ready when the other is. It creates an environment of opportunity for its recipient, which can be exploited for his own purpose when and where he so wishes. The display of recipiency, on the other hand, creates within the environment of free-floating opportunity a specific moment and location for its recipient to respond with an action. It declares an interest in receiving a response, a response in immediate juxtaposition to the display. It elicits an action and creates a location for its occurrence.

In the fragments at hand, the displays of availability and recipiency capture two rather different ways in which interactants may reengage talk and move out of silence. In each fragment the patient and doctor during the silence are orientated towards an appropriate and relevant next move: in the openings, movement into the business of the consultation; in Fragment 2:5, minimally some comment by the doctor on the patient's complaint. It is an environment of expectation, where a particular party, the doctor, is treated as responsible for the next activity. It is in this environment of potential talk that the display of recipiency can serve to encourage or push another to speak, eliciting a vocalization in response to a look. The display of recipiency allows one person to encourage another to begin activity without speaking or initiating the activity himself.

A display of recipiency can also serve to begin an encounter. For example in some video recordings of reception counters it is found that clients not only make themselves available but repeatedly turn towards the receptionists in an attempt to gain their attention. The length of the interval between successive looks provides just enough space to determine whether the desired response is forthcoming from the other. Moreover subsequent gaze shifts may be exaggerated, the whole head swinging away and back to underline the shift of orientation (see for example Fragment 4:5). If these attempts fail, then upgraded devices are used, such as waves[9] and in some cases vocalizations. Moreover one discerns from public commentary and the ethnographic literature that certain forms of street life and so-called deviant occupations rely upon persons not only making themselves available to others but also eliciting responses from "strangers" through a look. Simply turning and looking at another can serve to initiate interaction, yet has the advantage of avoiding a vocal commitment, which as a first move can lead to comment, complaint, and even prosecution. A display of recipiency encourages another to begin the activity without demanding his or her participation. As Goffman suggests, ". . . the initiator's first glance can be sufficiently tentative and ambiguous to allow him to act as if no initiation has been intended, if it appears that his overture is not desired" (1963/1966, p. 92).

In these examples and the fragments drawn from the beginning of the consultation, the response elicited by the display of recipiency serves to pass the floor back to the original party to conduct an activity. At reception counters for example, given some acknowledgement by the receptionist (which itself can be a shift of gaze towards the other), the patient is provided with the opportunity to disclose why he is there. Similarly, by encouraging the doctor to begin the business at hand, the patient receives the floor to disclose why he has come or how he is. In such cases turning towards another can work to gain the floor for some activity, the display of recipiency and its response serving as a prefatory device to an activity's production, the display of recipiency itself securing a recipient.

The opportunity provided through a display of recipiency may of course be declined. Turning and looking at another commits neither party to actually beginning but rather encourages a co-participant to cooperate in the start of an activity. Another's gaze, unlike, say, his utterance, can be ignored and the expected response withheld. Declining the opportunity afforded through a display of recipiency frequently involves one or both of the following forms of response. In receiving the gaze of another but not cooperating in the start of an activity, an interactant will turn further away, not infrequently shielding the eyes with the hand. Declinations to a display of recipiency are also a location for self-preens and other bodily focused activity;[10] in particular face and head touching. Consequently turning and looking at another does not leave the interactional environment untouched. They implicate a response and project relevancies for a certain location; whether it is accepted or declined, the recipient of another's gaze is responding to pressure generated by another through a slight, yet significant, shift in his visual orientation.

In the fragments discussed above, realigning gaze towards another serves as a first move out of silence and into talk and a mutual focus of involvement. The display of recipiency elicits an utterance and is prefatory to the start of an activity. A display of recipiency can occur within the course of talk and may itself be responsive to a preceding action.

Withholding an utterance and recipient action

<u>**Fragment 2:6   Transcript 1**</u>

```
Dr:     Do sit down::n
        (5.5)
Dr:     What's up:?
        (4.8)
P:      I've had a bad eye::: °(in there)=
Dr:     =oh: yeah
        (1.2)
P:      an:: it (had) fat flew up
```

Like many of the earlier instances, this is drawn from the beginning of a consultation. The doctor initiates the business with "Whats up:?" and the patient replies with "I've had a bad eye::: °(in there)=." Even though the doctor has asked the patient a question and initiated the business at hand, the patient's reply is delayed for nearly five seconds. The first second or so of the gap is occupied with the patient landing in the chair; from there on, however, he remains still, orientated towards the doctor and silent.

Fragment 2:6 Transcript 2

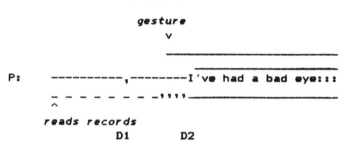

```
                       gesture
                         v
                  _____
                  _____
P:      ----------,--------I've had a bad eye:::
        _ _ _ _ _ _ _ _ _,''''_____
        ^
   reads records
              D1          D2
```

Drawings 1 and 2

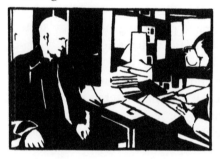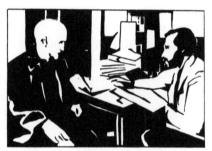

As the patient sits in the chair and is ready to reply, he is faced with a potential recipient who is reading the medical record cards. Four seconds or more into the gap, the doctor begins to turn from the records to the patient. The moment his gaze arrives at the patient's face, the patient begins to speak, replying to the doctor's question and cooperating in beginning the consultation proper. The doctor initiates the business of the consultation, but the patient withholds his reply and engagement in the activity until the doctor displays recipiency.

We enter the following consultation as the patient is describing the symptoms of his illness.

Fragment 2:7   Transcript 1

```
P:      I can't sleep
        (.)
Dr:     yeah
        (.)
P:      I've got a continuous stabbing headache
Dr:     yeahhh
        (1.2)
Dr:     yeah
P:      Well
        (1.4)
P:      this morning I (lost:: (.)down) until a quarter
        three
        (.3)
Dr:     yeah
P:      two o'clock the night before(.)just cannot sleep
```

Following "stabbing headache" and its receipt there is a silence; the doctor then utters "yeahhh" and turns towards the records. Rather than cooperating in the production of a lapse in the talk, the patient utters "Well," pauses, and then continues with a description of the difficulties he is suffering. The patient's "Well" appears to be positioned with respect to the doctor's turning away and serves to project that the patient has more to say; thus the 1.4-second gap is a pause within the patient's talk projecting an upcoming utterance rather than a warranted silence between the participants.

Drawings 1 and 2

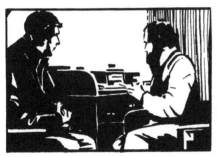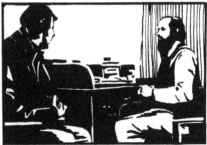

```
P:      Well----------,----this morning I (lost:::(.)
            D1              D2
```

As with the previous example, the patient's utterance is coordinated with the gaze of the potential recipient. The patient withholds the projected utterance until the doctor turns from the records and looks at the patient, the appropriate next speaker.

Unlike the examples in Fragments 2:6 and 2:7 where the patient withholds a relevant next utterance until the doctor looks up from the records, in the following example the speaker begins an utterance and then pauses prior to its completion.

Fragment 2:8   Transcript 1

```
Dr:    and they help(.)at the ti:me
       (.5)
P:     yeh (o.kay)
       (1.5)
P:     but I haven:'t (1.2) he gave me seven to take it
       dow: ┌:(n)
Dr:         │mm huh
       (.)  └
P:     taking them like that::t
```

As the patient continues with "but I haven:t" the doctor is reading the medical record cards. One second into the pause he begins to look up towards the patient. The moment his gaze arrives at her face she continues her utterance.

Fragment 2:8   Transcript 2

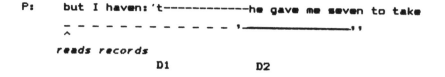

```
P:    but I haven:'t------------he gave me seven to take
      - - - - - - - - - - - - -'―――――――――'
           ^
      reads records
                     D1                  D2
```

Drawings 1 and 2

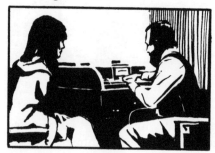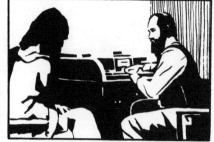

In each instance therefore an utterance within an environment of talk is coordinated with the nonvocal behaviour of the potential recipient. The speaker withholds a reply or pauses within the articulation of an utterance until the cointeractant has turned his gaze towards – displayed recipiency to – the speaker. The production of the speech occurs in immediate juxtaposition to the realignment of the recipient's gaze. As in the earlier examples, it is as if turning towards the speaker encourages the production of talk, the relevant next action.

Unlike the earlier examples, however, this example shows that the realignment of gaze by the cointeractant, the display of recipiency, may itself be responsive to a preceding action. In Fragment 2:6 the patient withholds a sequentially relevant next action, an answer to the doctor's question. In the following instance the patient projects more to follow and then delays its production. And in the last example the speaker begins an utterance and pauses prior to its completion. In each case the speaker or potential speaker encourages recipient activity by pausing and withholding the sequentially relevant or projected action (cf. C. Goodwin 1979a, 1980, 1981a; Jefferson 1983a). Withholding an utterance or part of the utterance encourages the potential recipient to realign his gaze towards the speaker and display recipiency to the activities of the speaker. In contrast to the examples discussed earlier, here the display of recipiency is the pivotal action in a three-action sequence.[11] The pause encourages the potential recipient to realign his gaze, and the realignment of gaze encourages the production or continuation of the utterance. Thus the utterance is coordinated with the visual behaviour of the potential recipient, the speaker withholding talk until the cointeractant has realigned his gaze and displayed recipiency to the speaker.

The display of recipiency is of course intimately related to the focus of a person's attention. In encouraging another to turn towards you whilst you are speaking, you are not simply asking to be looked at but to receive some indication that your co-participant is attending to and receiving the activity in hand. Turning towards another is a way of displaying recipiency, showing attention, without interrupting the activity in which the other is engaged. This link between the direction of a person's gaze and the focus of his attention permeates social life and has formed the foundation of numerous works and studies both in the arts and human sciences. Taking a small but important collection of studies of communication – for example Atkinson 1984; Austin 1806; Darwin 1872; Fisher, Munty, and Senders 1981; Goffman 1963, 1967; C. Goodwin 1981a; Kendon 1967; Scheflen 1973 – we find the tie between gaze and attention informing a range of empirical findings. Argyle and Cook neatly capture the point in question:

> People who notice when others are looking at them or who are aware of how much someone is looking, will probably draw some inference from this behaviour. The first and simplest inference is that the other is attending to them.

> Glances are used by listeners to indicate continual attention and willingness to listen. Aversion of gaze means lack of interest or disapproval. (1976, pp. 84, 121)

Thus it seems reasonable to suggest that when faced with a potential recipient who is looking at the medical records, a speaker might well infer that his partner's attention lies in the papers within his regard. Consequently a speaker may withhold talk until he secures evidence that the cointeractant is prepared to attend to the utterance and activity. And in withholding a sequentially appropriate or projected utterance the speaker can encourage the potential recipient to realign his gaze and refocus attention, delaying talk until the services of a recipient are forthcoming. Thus in turning towards another and displaying recipiency, an interactant can show the focus of his attention and involvement; the display of recipiency and showing attention go hand in hand.[12]

Recipient selection and collaborative lookings

The examples discussed so far have all been drawn from dyadic consultations involving just a doctor and patient. In interaction involving more than two persons gaze may be used to differentiate the co-participants and feature in the selection of a potential recipient and next speaker. The following captures a particularly complex stretch of action and will be examined in detail, step by step.

Fragment 2:9   Transcript 1

```
Dr:    an his name is?er:,
M:     Rob James
       (.2)
Dr:    Rob
       (.7)
Dr:    O.kay: Rob (.6) hhhOhh (.3)
Dr:    hhh(.)hhhhhhOhhhhh(.)(slap)(.2)hhhhhhhhh(.3)
M:     ur: ⌈n:::::::::
Dr:        ⌊don't look too happy today
M:     heehh
Dr:    whats:er:: matter
M:     Ohhhh I was wanting something for his coughing
```

The fragment is drawn from the beginning of a consultation in which a mother presents the illness of her young child Rob. After an exchange through which the doctor checks the identity of the patient, the doctor utters "O.kay: Rob," an utterance which receives no immediate response from either the child or his mother.[13] This is followed by various gaps, inbreaths, and outbreaths, with finally the child's mother beginning to speak. As she speaks the doctor enters in overlap with a comment about Rob, and the mother laughs. The doctor then initiates the business of the consultation and receives a report of Rob's recent illness. Visually it is an intriguing stretch of interaction; we will begin its explication where the doctor attempts to start the ball rolling with "O.kay: Rob."

Fragment 2:9   Transcript 2

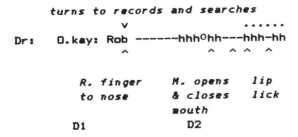

Drawings 1 and 2

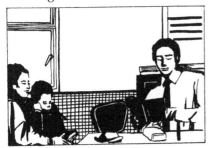 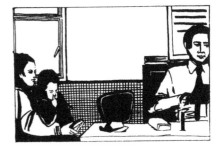

The doctor utters "O.kay: Rob" as he lands in the chair opposite his fellow participants. The utterance vocalizes the doctor's availability, his readiness to begin, and selects Rob as the appropriate respondent. Yet neither Rob nor his mother replies to the doctor, and the only response to the utterance is that Rob's finger pops straight up his nose. Given some of the points raised earlier it is not surprising that the doctor receives no reply. As he vocalizes his readiness, he simultaneously turns and faces the opposite direction, undertaking a search for his young patient's records. The potential speakers, both Rob and his mum, are faced with a candidate recipient who is visibly involved in another activity.

The mother does in fact make a couple of attempts to speak but then backs down. Twice whilst the doctor is looking for the records she opens her mouth and takes in air as if preparing to speak. This preparatory behaviour, rather like revving up at the lights, coincides with the doctor withdrawing records and beginning to turn around towards his co-participants. As he discovers they are the wrong records, he thrusts his hand back into the pile, and his cointeractant abandons her first attempt to speak, simply closing her mouth. As he begins to turn round for the second time, the mother takes in air as if to speak, yet as his face enters view she abandons her preparation, producing an elaborate lick of her lips.

Fragment 2:9   Transcript 3

```
      turns round
      closed eyes, gripped mouth
      v
      . . . . . . . . . . _____
Dr:   hhh-hhhhhhOhhhhh-(slam)
M:    _____. . . . ._____
      Dr            Rob
      D3            D4
```

Drawings 3 and 4

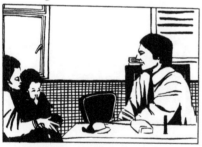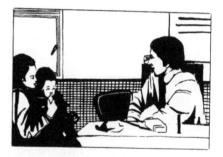

As the doctor turns round, and before he enters the view of his fellow participants, he grips his mouth and squeezes his eyes tight. In this way the doctor shows that he is not taking the opportunity to speak, an opportunity afforded through his own movement into availability. He turns, retaining his facial expression past the mother, and opens his eyes as he nears Rob; he displays recipiency to the child, selecting Rob as the party who should speak next.

In closing his eyes the doctor is able to bypass a cointeractant to enable him to encourage a particular party to speak next, and the mother cooperates by abandoning her preparation to speak and producing a lick of the lips.[14] However, the mother does not simply cooperate in the attempt to encourage Rob to speak by withholding talk herself, but actively collaborates with the doctor. As the doctor swings round, the mother imitates his facial expression and turns towards her son. Gripping her mouth and looking at the child, the mother joins forces with her fellow interactant in order to elicit a response from Rob. This collaborative display of recipiency fails to encourage Rob to respond either vocally or nonvocally, and he continues to gaze at the desk, remaining quite still. The doctor slams the records on the desk.

Fragment 2:9 Transcript 4

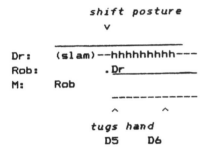

Drawings 5 and 6

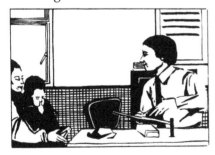
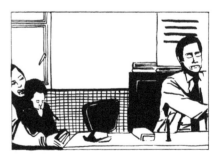

Rob remains unmoved. Continuing to gaze at the child, the mother and doctor drop their gripped mouths. On slamming the records the doctor turns to one side, and finally this slight movement meets with some success. Rob turns and looks at the doctor, yet still remains silent.

It will be recalled that at the beginning of this encounter Rob's finger went up his nose, and in consequence his hand covered his mouth.

There it remains throughout the fragment thus far. As the participants continue to display recipiency to Rob, his mother tries to remove his hand from his mouth and finger from his nose, attempting to deal with any obstacles that might be interfering with his ability to speak to the doctor. She tries twice to remove the child's hand; following the failure of the second attempt with still no vocalization from Rob, the mother herself begins to speak. Her utterance ("ur:n::::::::") is content-free. It neither commits itself to beginning the business of the consultation nor remarks on Rob's behaviour. It invites the doctor to speak, and this he does, entering in overlap with a joke about Rob and his sullenness. Following the mother's laugh the doctor successfully initiates the business of the consultation.

One additional comment: The way in which Rob's mother attempts to remove his hand is curious and not surprisingly fails. Rather than place her hand over his and push it down, as she does a little later – removing the hand with little difficulty – she takes Rob's wrist and attempts to pull it down and away from his chin. Perhaps the action is produced in this fashion to avoid the consequences of placing her hand on top of Rob's. Had she done this, she would not only have placed her hand across the line of the participant's mutual regard and disrupted, if only temporarily, the doctor's display of recipiency, but also inadvertently placed her hand over Rob's mouth, adding to his difficulties in speaking. In fashioning the gesture as she does, the mother continues to collaborate with the doctor, assisting his attempts to elicit a response from the child with his continued looking.

In this brief segment of interaction, lasting only a few seconds, there are numerous attempts to elicit a response from Rob. The vocalized availability fails, and its failure is followed by collaborative displays of recipiency. Their failure to elicit a response finds the doctor slamming the records, and its failure leads to subsequent displays of recipiency. A posture shift by the doctor successfully elicits Rob's gaze, but speech is not forthcoming. Following the failure of the slam of records, the mother again collaborates with the doctor: She holds her display of recipiency on Rob, concurrently attempting to remove his hand from his mouth, a possible hindrance to his responding. As we know, all fail.

Two persons, then, are engaged in eliciting a response from a third. Each attempt generates an interactional slot where an appropriate response from the third party is relevant. On its failure to occur, a further attempt is made, and so on. Each attempt occurs within the developing history of the interaction. A subsequent attempt, following a failure, is not merely trying another, but rather choosing what might succeed, given

what has failed so far. The sequential structure of the displays of recipiency allows the doctor and mother to discern the absence of a response
and build their case accordingly. Each display of recipiency and every
action by the doctor and the mother are delicately and precisely organized
to elicit a response at some point in the developing course of the interaction. The actions of the mother and the doctor are designed with respect
to the contingencies that have arisen so far and the possible local, interactional solutions to the problems they are facing. Thus this small
segment involves a constant shifting, a negotiation in which repeated
attempts at eliciting talk mainly through looking at another are coordinated by the participants with regard to the local interactional history.

Discussion and remarks on the beginning of the consultation

The power of the look features in human communication and interaction.
Even without looking at the person who is looking at one, a person is
aware that he is falling under the gaze of another. Being looked at renders
one the object of another's attention; it shows that one is being taken
account of in some fashion and that one may be subject to the expectations of another. Becoming the focus of another's attention renders a
person relevant to his action and activity, as featuring here and now in
his concerns and matters at hand. The look affects the other; it can arouse
and encourage activity, initiate or progress interaction between persons.
Turning and looking at another is used in human interaction; it accomplishes particular work or tasks, performs actions and activities.

In the examples discussed here, we find the realignment of gaze coupled at times with a postural reorientation used to display recipiency,
to show that one is attentive to and expects to receive something from
another. The display of recipiency is interactionally coordinated and sequentially implicative. It is elicitive, it generates an interactional location,
immediately following its occurrence where another is encouraged and
constrained to respond, to produce a next action or activity. In the earlier
fragments for example, within an environment of open opportunity
where movement into the business of the consultation is an appropriate
next move, the display of recipiency encourages the doctor to speak and
initiate talk on topic and thereby elicit the patient's reason for the visit.
As a first action, the display of recipiency provides an opportunity and
position for an action or activity by another and allows an interactant to
inspect what immediately follows in order to discern how the other is
managing the object. The sequential structure of a display of recipiency
and its response is such that, as in Fragment 2:9, interactants may make

repeated attempts to elicit an action from another through a display of recipiency, given the recognizable absence of particular responses in certain locations. Thus however slight or seemingly unnoticeable, the display of recipiency is sequentially and interactionally organized, and its relevancies are used and orientated to by participants in actual situations.

A display of recipiency may occur as a second action, itself a response to a preceding action or activity. A speaker can withhold a sequentially relevant utterance or pause within the course of its articulation and successfully encourage the potential recipient to realign his gaze. In such cases the utterance itself is a product of the interaction between the participants and is sensitive to the speaker's requirements and the state of the recipient's participation in the activity. As a second action, a response to the pause, the display of recipiency forms a pivot between an elicitation of recipient activity and the production of talk. The display of recipiency simultaneously responds to a preceding action and encourages the articulation of an utterance. In encouraging the potential recipient to realign his gaze, the speaker commits himself to respond and produce a particular action or activity. The display of recipiency operates retroactively and proactively, dealing with an immediately prior action and eliciting a next.

Whether the first or second action within a sequence, in the examples discussed here (save those in Fragments 2:5 and 2:9) the display of recipiency forms part of a package which prefaces a subsequent action or activity.[15] In the fragments drawn from the beginnings of consultations the display of recipiency encourages the doctor to initiate talk on topic, and the doctor's utterance passes the floor back to the patient, providing the opportunity to disclose the reason for the visit or how the patient is feeling. The display of recipiency and the doctor's topic-initiating utterance serve as a two-action sequence through which the patient gains the floor to talk about his complaint over a consecutive series of utterances. In other fragments the display of recipiency occasions the production or continuation of an activity by the other, the pause and realignment of gaze providing a suitable environment for the articulation of the business or topic at hand. In both collections of examples therefore the display of recipiency is part of a two-action sequence which sets the scene and provides the opportunity for the production of an activity which forms part of the mainstream of the topic and business of the interaction.

At the beginning of the medical consultation it is the doctor who typically produces the utterance which begins talk on topic, the business of the consultation. This is not insignificant in the structure of the consultation and the work of diagnosis and prognosis. The consultation has a characteristic social organization, an interview structure that entails a chain (cf. Sacks 1972b) or series of interrelated questions and answers which provide a vehicle for the disclosure and elicitation of the patient's complaint and/or its present condition, and thereby its prognosis and management. Under the guise of questions and answers a range of activities are accomplished in the consultation, yet the doctor typically initiates each sequence, and if necessary interrupts the patient in the course of his or her reply for clarification and the like. This apparent formal character of the consultation relies upon the doctor initiating the business at hand and mutually establishing with the patient the interview structure of the consultation from the beginning, where the patient provides his reason for the visit or details of how he is.

Initiating the business of the consultation not only allows the doctor to set in motion the interview structure of the consultation but also to tailor the actual beginning for the particular patient. The utterances which initiate talk on topic, for example "Whats up:?" (Fragment 2:6) and "Ho-wav:: you bee:n:" (Fragment 2:3), are designed, often on the basis of information gathered from the medical records, for this patient on this occasion. The utterances display the state of knowledge the doctor has concerning the patient's complaint, whether he is familiar with the problem and its details, as in a return appointment, or ignorant of the reason for the visit. The topic-initiating utterance allows the patient to know before actually beginning what needs to be told and what can be left unsaid; to design the description of his complaint to what the doctor knows about this patient's illness. Were the patient to begin the business at hand, he would be ignorant of what and how much to tell, especially on return visits to the doctor.

It has been seen that in the preliminaries of the consultation both doctor and patient prepare for the business at hand – a stretch of continuous activity which necessitates their coordination and joint attention. Besides the various vocal exchanges, they achieve a suitable spatial and physical alignment, and the doctor arranges his desk and reads the medical record cards. The doctor is able to discern when the patient is physically available and ready to begin, frequently withholding the start of business until the patient has sat down and assumed a face-to-face orientation. The patient on the other hand is often unable to tell whether the doctor has dealt with all the preliminary matters necessary to beginning the consultation proper; for example whether he has gathered enough information from the medical record cards or finished dealing with the written particulars of the last patient. The patient's availability is clearly visible;

but for the doctor the arrival of the next case marks just another moment in a state of continuous activity.

There are therefore distinct practical advantages in the fact that the doctor typically initiates talk on topic, the business at hand. The patient's display of both availability and recipiency preserves the opportunity for the doctor to begin the proceedings. The display of availability, as in the first example, provides the doctor with a stretch of undifferentiated opportunity to begin wherever he wishes. The display of recipiency encourages the doctor to produce action at a certain moment; it encourages and sets a location for response. However, though the display of recipiency might encourage the co-participant to begin, it commits neither party to actually beginning; no vocalization is produced, no response demanded. The display of recipiency pushes the other to begin whilst not interrupting the activity in which he is engaged; it does not undermine the doctor's opportunity actually to begin the business at hand when he is ready and so desires. The display of recipiency respects a formal and practical characteristic of the consultation and plays a small but important part in preserving its structural organization. It also perhaps bears tribute to and reproduces the momentary categorical membership of the participants: a patient requesting but not demanding the attention of a doctor.

3. Maintaining involvement in the consultation

The task of becoming spontaneously involved in something
when it is a duty to oneself or others to do so, is a ticklish thing,
as we all know from experience with dull chores or threatening
ones. The individual's actions must happen to satisfy his
involvement obligations, but in a certain sense he cannot act in
order to satisfy these obligations, for such an effort would
require him to shift his attention from the topic of conversation
to the problem of being spontaneously involved in it. Here, in a
component of non-rational impulsiveness–not only tolerated but
actually demanded–we find an important way in which the
interactional order differs from other kinds of social order.

Goffman 1967/1972, p. 155

There is nothing so brutally shocking, nor so little forgiven, as
a seeming inattention to the person who is speaking to you: and
I have known many a man knocked down for (in my opinion) a
much slighter provocation than that shocking inattention which I
mean. I have seen many people who, while you are speaking to
them, instead of looking at, and attending you, fix their eyes
upon the ceiling, or some other part of the room, look out the
window, play with a dog, twirl their snuff box, or pick their
nose. Nothing discovers a little, futile frivolous mind more than
this, and nothing is so offensively ill-bred; it is an explicit
declaration on your part that every, the most trifling, object
deserves your attention more than all that can be said by the
person who is speaking to you. . . . Be therefore, I beg of you,
not only really, but seemingly and manifestly, attentive to
whoever speaks to you. . . .

Lord Chesterfield (1752) 1984, pp. 261–2

The medical consultation, like other forms of social interaction, requires
the participants to sustain some semblance of mutual involvement in
the business or topic at hand. The participants are obliged to speak, to
disclose complaints, to offer forms of management and the like, and to
display attention to and show an appreciation of the activities and actions
of their co-participants. This semblance of mutual involvement has to

49

be continually maintained and can shift within the course of a single utterance from a seeming lack of interest to deep engrossment in the matters at hand. Yet as Goffman (1967) points out, sustaining involvement is a delicate affair; if it were addressed explicitly by the participants it would shift the focus of attention from the business of the consultation to the problem of being involved in it.

The medical consultation is particularly interesting when addressing the problem of involvement in social interaction. For example, unlike many forms of human interaction, the consultation requires a curious fluidity of involvement, a continual shifting between various concerns, be they in the foreground or the background of the participants' attention. Thus, as well as conversing with the patient, the doctor engages in a myriad of other activities in the patient's presence, including conducting physical examinations, reading and writing the medical record cards, and issuing prescriptions, sick notes and the like. These concerns may be dealt with in distinct phases of the consultation, though more frequently they are conducted alongside the flow of talk between the patient and the doctor. For the doctor and the patient, involvement has to be sustained in the face of simultaneous and often competing demands.

The medical consultation also requires one participant to generate an "objective" assessment of the state of health of another, an assessment that is used to warrant certain types of treatment: access to drugs, leave from work, and the various rights and responsibilities associated with the sick role. The decisions of the medical practitioner are in large part formed in the light of what the patient, or someone on behalf of the patient, says during the consultation. Recent studies in conversation analysis have demonstrated how a speaker's talk is thoroughly bound up with behaviour of the recipient (see for example C. Goodwin 1979a, 1980, 1981a; Heath 1984a, b; Jefferson 1980, 1983b), and hence how the doctor attends to and participates in the patient's talk may be consequential to what the patient says, medical decision making, treatment programmes, and the like.

In a rather different vein, we have with the medical consultation an example of a certain form of occupational activity which, though routine and repetitive, requires a high degree of involvement and precise attention to detail. The doctor maintains involvement across a range of cases, dealt with in relatively brief interactions which include a wide diversity of co-participants drawn from very different backgrounds. Intuitively one might expect that the nature of the occupational activity coupled with the wide diversity of participants may have a significant influence on the maintenance of involvement in the consultation.

This and the following couple of chapters explore the fashion in which patient and doctor sustain involvement during the medical consultation and the ways in which they participate in and attend to each other's actions and activities. The concern of this chapter is to examine how gestures and other forms of body movement are employed to encourage others to attend and to show how talk is synchronized with the nonvocal actions of both the speaker and the recipient. Of particular interest is the design of visual action and the ways in which the minutiae of human movement – a gesture, a tug, a shift in posture – are carefully shaped with respect to the context at hand and the interactional tasks the movement is performing. The design of human movement casts light on the problem of sustaining involvement and is perhaps relevant to a classic issue in sociological analysis, the integration of individuals in interaction and society.[1]

There are of course a host of ways in which the issues of sustaining involvement in the medical consultation might be addressed. The focus here is on the interactional coordination of visual and vocal behaviour, and the examples are selected to capture a variety of participants attempting to establish each other's attention. It should be mentioned, however, that within the data corpus of medical interviews there is a preponderance towards patient- or client-initiated attempts to gain the attention of the doctor or professional. This is not simply because patients or clients have to hold the floor to disclose their complaints over successive utterances and thereby might run into difficulties of holding the other's attention, but rather that special issues arise in professional conduct which compete for the practitioners' attention. These aspects will be dealt with in more detail in Chapter 7; the concern here is to explore aspects of the social organization which enable people to maintain involvement in the medical consultation and perhaps other forms of face-to-face interaction.

Establishing a recipient through body movement

Besides pauses, there are other ways in which a person might encourage another to realign his or her gaze.

Fragment 3:1 Transcript 1

```
(20.00) ((Dr writes prescription throughout))
F:  Allright (.2) Ohhhhh he got(.)two children like you
    (1.2)
Dr: Yes(.)I have
F:  Yerse because°hh (.2)erm::: see::........
```

This utterance is spoken during a lengthy silence as the doctor writes a prescription for his two young patients Lythia and Asia. The utterance is spoken by their father, who is standing behind his two seated daughters. As he begins the utterance proper "he got . . ." the father waves his hand up and down by the side of the face of his younger daughter, Lythia. The gesture appears to catch her eye, and she turns from the doctor to the face of her father. As her gaze arrives at the speaker he drops his hand and abandons the gesture.

Fragment 3:1   Drawings 1 and 2

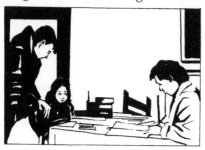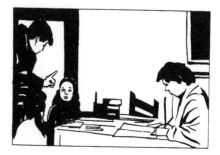

D1   D2

P: Alright--ᴼhhhhh he got-two children like you

The gesture is not the first attempt by the speaker to secure the gaze of the potential recipient. Earlier in the utterance, actually before he begins to speak, the father takes hold of his daughter's shoulder and begins to peer round towards her face. As his hand lands on the shoulder, the speaker attempts to tug his daughter towards him, but she steadfastly continues looking at the doctor. He tries again, pulling her shoulder further back, but as before her gaze remains firmly on the doctor. On receiving no response to the second tug, the speaker abandons his daughter's shoulder and begins to wave his hand up and down; she realigns her gaze, and he ceases all gestural activity.

Fragment 3:1 Transcript 2

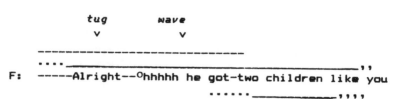

In the following couple of examples, as in Fragment 3:1, a speaker in the course of an utterance successfully elicits the gaze of the potential recipient through movement. We enter the first example as the patient begins to voice his elation on concluding his finals whilst the doctor writes his prescription.

Fragment 3:2 Transcript 1

```
     (3.4)
P:   It's worth going through just to have this wonderful
     period of absolutely doing noth:ing(.)it's
     marvellous
     (1.0)
Dr:  Som[e people feel so fla:t at the end of it
        [eh
```

Drawings 1 and 2

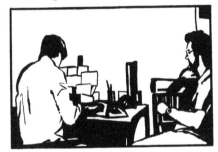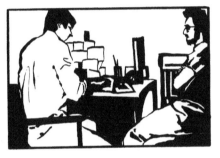

```
         D1                        D2
P:   this wonderful period of absolutely doing nothing(.)
```

It can be seen from the drawings that the patient changes his position and the doctor turns from the desk to the speaker. Near the beginning of the utterance the patient throws himself back into the chair and stretches his arms over his shoulders as if to scratch his back. The movement fails to attract the other's notice; and the doctor continues to write. Following a brief gap, the patient once again starts the move, this time moving posturally to one side, nearing the doctor's area of focus. As he moves, the doctor looks up from the desk and turns towards the speaker. The speaker secures the gaze of the recipient towards the end of the utterance and it is as if the additional component "it's marvellous," reemphasizing the elation, is tagged on in light of the doctor's shift in alignment. However, though the patient successfully secures a response from the doctor, he does not appear to secure the recipient's agreement. The reply undercuts a little of the patient's elation, and as the doctor speaks he returns once more to writing the prescription.

The next fragment contains a number of examples of the way in which a realignment of gaze may be coordinated with another's body movement.

Fragment 3:3 Transcript 1

```
Dr:    You see I don't think theres any sign of anything
       broken(.)if ┌:: there is there is a break in the
                   └no::
Dr:    collar bone(.2) °hh the only treatment is ┌support
P:                                                └yes
Dr:    (.)for a week or two and then it settles ┘
       <but ┌I think
P:          └yes
Dr:    you've got eh flare up(.)°hh in the joint(.)that
       between the collarbone and the breast bone ┌::
P:                                                 └mmm
Dr:     hhh(.)an::: (.8)it ┌would be better:: hooo ┌ps::s
P:                         └(erm)                  └sorry
Dr:    shes away hhh(.)heh heh heh hhh°hhh(.)come on
       girlie(.)you're adventurous
```

Throughout much of this fragment the baby daughter of the patient is playing havoc in the corner of the surgery. As the doctor offers his advice, the patient makes successive attempts to fetch the troublemaker and rescue the consulting room. The baby's activities pass unnoticed by the doctor, and the mother's attempts to break away are treated like the behaviour of a recalcitrant recipient, rather than of a person who is attempting to save the surgery from destruction. The following transcripts capture just a couple of the occasions in which the mother attempts to disengage from the talk of the doctor and deal with her baby.

Fragment 3:3 Transcript 2

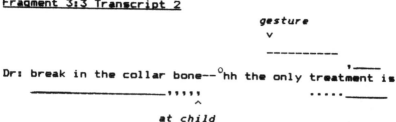

Fragment 3:3 Transcript 3

```
                                gesture
                                   v
                           --------
                                                    ----
Dr: then it settles<but I think you've got eh flare up
    _____,,,,              ....._____
                         ^
             at child
```

In both cases the mother turns her gaze to the child and begins to stand. As she begins to break away, the doctor continues speaking and simultaneously begins to gesture. In both cases the doctor clasps his stomach as if in pain. And as the doctor's hand moves towards his stomach the patient turns back towards the speaker, abandoning her attempt to deal with the baby. The patient's realignment is coordinated with the doctor's gestural activity, each gesture of the speaker serving to realign the gaze and occupation of the potential recipient. As for the surgery, the doctor learns the hard way.

In the same way that a person may wave to catch the eye of a cabby or auctioneer, or a conductor thrust the baton to gain the attention of a particular musician,[2] so a speaker in face-to-face interactions may elicit another's gaze through a nonvocal action. In each example we find the speaker faced with a potential recipient who is visibly engaged elsewhere. The speakers seek to have some demonstration that the potential recipient is prepared to receive or is actually engaged in receiving the utterance(s). The speakers are in search of attention and attempting to establish the co-occurring talk as the primary involvement, the business or topic at hand. The speaker uses visual action to encourage the cointeractant to cooperate and participate in the activity, the recipient's realignment of gaze providing evidence during the course of the utterance that it is being received. In seeking the cointeractant's attention, the speaker attempts to secure the sequential and interactional significance of his talk.

Even in the few examples presented so far, it is found that speakers use a wide variety of movements to elicit another's gaze, ranging from tugging a shoulder through to clutching one's stomach. In its particular context each movement serves to perform a similar type of action, encouraging the cointeractant to turn towards the face of the speaker. The movements are sequentially implicative; they project an appropriate next action, an action which should occur in a particular position, immediately following the first. Eliciting gaze through body movement is a tightly ordered, sequentially organized two-action sequence, the first encouraging a particular form of response from another.[3] Consequently the speaker is able to inspect particular positions within the interaction in order to determine whether the appropriate action has been performed by the potential recipient. If the appropriate response is not immediately forthcoming, as in Fragment 3:1 and perhaps Fragment 3:2, the speaker can undertake remedial action, producing successive movements in an attempt to encourage another to realign his gaze and display recipiency. Successive attempts may entail not simply the original movement being recycled, but more often a reshaping of the original or even a different form of movement altogether. The speaker recreates and refashions the action in the light of the local circumstances, moment by moment, in an attempt to make one succeed where others have failed.

In the preceding chapter it was observed how a speaker can encourage another to display recipiency by withholding interactionally relevant talk. A sequentially appropriate utterance might be delayed, or a speaker could pause within its articulation and thereby elicit the gaze and attention of the recipient. In the examples presented here we find the speaker employing visual action alongside the articulation of an utterance to establish the participation of a cointeractant, a display of recipiency, attention to the talk and business at hand. Unlike pauses either prior to or during the production of an utterance, the speaker's movements do not necessarily involve delaying the accompanying activity. The speaker produces the utterance, gathering the recipient's participation in its course; the movements occur alongside the utterance and do not render talk dependent upon a realignment of gaze by the other.[4] In one sense they are a more gentle attempt at encouraging the cointeractant to pay attention, at least in Fragments 3:2 and 3:3, encouraging but not demanding a reorientation from the recipient.

In many examples, however, the articulation of the utterance bears a close relation to the visual behaviour of the potential recipient(s) and the speaker.

Coordinating an utterance with the visual behaviour of both speaker and recipient

Before addressing a remark to another, a speaker may wish to have some indication that the candidate recipient is willing to attend.

<u>Fragment 3:4 Transcript 1</u>

```
SW:    and I will
       (.3)
M:     um
SW:    see him and tell him about this interview that
       we've had
M:     yes
SW:    together °hhhhh I think he will be able to prescribe
       something hhh
M:          yes
SW:    which Jennifer (.6) Jennifer (.3) you'll have to
       ta::ke Ohh (.3) regularly without let up
```

This fragment is drawn from a psychiatric-social-work interview in which
a mother discusses the difficulties she is having with her teenage daughter Jennifer. Jennifer is present during the interview but rarely participates
either as a speaker or hearer. As we enter the fragment we find the
interviewer telling the mother that she will discuss the interview with
her daughter's general practitioner. Jennifer is staring at the floor. As
she begins to discuss the management of the case, the psychiatric social
worker turns towards Jennifer and makes a vocal attempt to elicit a response with "which Jennifer." The vocalization is emphasized and coupled with a hand thrust towards the client—an exaggerated display of
recipiency. Jennifer remains still, continuing to stare at the floor, and
following a 0.6-second silence the interviewer makes a second attempt
to secure a response from her potential recipient. Towards the completion
of the second summons, Jennifer begins to shift her gaze from the floor
to the speaker. The moment her gaze arrives, the psychiatric social
worker produces the utterance "you'll have to . . . ," instructing Jennifer
concerning the proposed treatment.

Fragment 3:4   Drawings 1 and 2

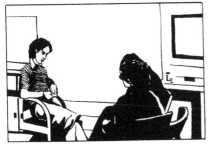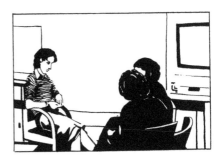

D1   D2

SW: which Jennifer (.6) Jennifer (.3) you'll have to ...

On an initial look at the data it is assumed that the second vocal summons, "Jennifer," secures the realignment of gaze by the recipient. Yet Jennifer turns towards the speaker at the end of "Jennifer" and has already ignored a previous summons accompanied by a head thrust. On closer inspection one notices a foot movement which begins in the gap between the two summonses. The interviewer's foot lands on the client's shin towards the end of the second "Jennifer," and as it touches the leg the client turns towards the speaker. The social worker encourages Jennifer to realign her gaze by tapping her shin, and in displaying recipiency to the speaker Jennifer encourages the production of the utterance.

In some cases a speaker may withhold talk within the articulation of an utterance until he has received a display of recipiency from a cointeractant.

Fragment 3:5   Transcript 1

```
Dr:    Now you've mentioned there were three problems
       have we discussed two of them?
       (.7)
P:     Well no(.)only that when I get these feelings erm:
       ::I end up wither (.3)°all:::mi:ghty: headache
       (.3)
P:     and what I was going to ask was can I have some
       distalgesics.
```

After dealing with two of the patient's problems the doctor asks about the third. As the patient begins to reply the doctor turns and reads the medical record cards. At "I end" the patient begins a gesture. She forms her hand into a point and begins a circular motion, widening its circumference as the utterance progresses. At "wither" she thrusts the pointing hand towards the doctor.

Fragment 3:5   Transcript 2

```
       start       thrust
         v           v
       ---------------------
P:     I end up wither---all:::mi:ghty: headache

       - - - - - - - _···▪_____
       ^reads records
```

The speaker pauses within the course of the utterance and awaits the arrival of the gaze of the potential recipient. The moment the doctor looks at the patient, she produces the description of her suffering "all:::mi:ghty: headache." It is said with an exaggerated pronunciation at low volume, almost whispered to the recipient. It not only describes the complaint but, coupled with a facial expression the patient adopts, captures in the way it is produced actual suffering. It is as if in describing her complaint the patient momentarily suffers its symptoms.[5] From the beginning of the utterance the patient looks as if she is attempting to gain the doctor's attention. The gesture with its successively widening circumference is designed to elicit his gaze, and when all else fails the speaker thrusts the pointing finger towards the doctor. The speaker begins the utterance attempting to gather the participation of the recipient along its course; on finding the doctor continuing to read the records she withholds the final and crucial component of the utterance until he has turned towards her. As his gaze arrives she produces the complaint for a seeing recipient.

Fragment 3:6 Transcript 1

```
        ((knocks))
Dr:     Come in
        (1.5)
Dr:     Hello
P:      Hello
        (3.4)
Dr:     Err::(.)how are things Mister (.6) Arma⌈n?
P:                                          ⌊Erm:::(.5)
        all right(.)I just err::(1.0)come to (.7) have a
        look you know about err:::(.7) heerrr: (.4) have
        you got any information from hos:pital
Dr:     No::: (.3) I don't think so (.3) urm:::
```

This fragment is drawn from the beginning of a consultation. The doctor initiates the business at hand, and the patient begins to reply. The patient's reply runs into some difficulties; the speaker hesitates, pausing a number of times and producing "err:::s" as if delaying stating his reason for visiting the doctor. Within the utterance there is, however, a clear and unperturbed stretch of talk which brings the patient to the point of detailing his visit – "have a look you know about." Before it is complete the patient once again runs into trouble.

Fragment 3:6 Transcript 2

```
            posture shift
              leg cross

            -----

        _____,       ._____
P:      come to--------have a look you know about err:::
        _ _ _ _ _ _..·_____ ,,,,
        ^
        reads
        records
        D1              D2
```

As the patient begins to reply, the doctor is reading the medical record cards. Following "come to" the doctor turns from the records to the patient; the moment his gaze arrives, the patient produces "have a look you know about," the clear and unperturbed stretch of talk. At the word "know" the doctor begins to turn back to the records, and at that moment the speaker once more runs into trouble, producing "err:::" and pausing. Following the observations made in the preceding chapter concerning pauses and the findings made by C. Goodwin (1979a, 1980, 1981a), it is likely that the disfluencies in the initial part of the utterance are themselves attempts to elicit the gaze of the doctor. If so, they fail to encourage the recipient to realign his gaze, and in the pause following "come to" the patient crosses his legs. As his legs rise and he moves backwards, the doctor abandons the records and turns to the patient.

Fragment 3:6   Drawings 1 and 2

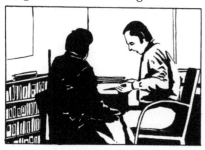 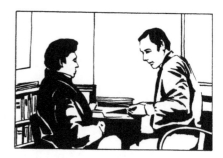

As in earlier examples, through a body movement the speaker successfully encourages the doctor to abandon the records and look up. The movement occurs within the utterance itself, deep in the course of its articulation. It follows earlier attempts produced through pauses and other disfluencies that serve to stall the production of the utterance, as if the speaker is attempting to gain the cointeractant's attention prior to providing the gist of the utterance. On successfully encouraging the other to pay attention, the patient articulates a clean stretch of talk and just at the moment of disclosure hesitates as he loses the gaze of the recipient.

In each instance the speaker is faced with a potential recipient who is visibly involved elsewhere and providing little evidence that he is prepared to attend to the utterance. In two of the examples it is the patient who, on speaking, finds the doctor reading the medical records; in the other instance a speaker, a psychiatric social worker, is faced by a recalcitrant client who provides little indication of involvement in the interview. In each case the speaker uses some form of body movement, a gesture, a posture shift, even a leg tap, to encourage the cointeractant to realign his or her gaze and display recipiency. The body movement serves to focus the participant's attention on the talk and, if only temporarily, establish the utterance as the primary involvement of the interview.

In contrast to earlier examples, the production of talk in each instance is synchronized with the visual behaviour of the potential recipient and the speaker. In Fragment 3:4 for example the interviewer withholds an utterance until she has successfully encouraged the client to turn towards her and display recipiency. In Fragments 3:5 and 3:6 we find the speaker, within the production of an utterance, delaying talk until the recipient abandons using the records and realigns his gaze. In each instance the speaker encourages the potential recipient to realign his gaze and display attention to the utterance through a body movement. The speaker's movement elicits the gaze of the cointeractant, and the realignment of gaze encourages the production of talk. These examples are not unlike those discussed in the previous chapter; we find a three-action sequence in which the speaker elicits gaze and gaze encourages talk, the display of recipiency serving as a pivoted action, operating retroactively and proactively. Thus the utterance is an interactional product, coordinated through the nonvocal actions of both speaker and recipient. The speaker uses body movement to establish an appropriate environment for an utterance, the movement and realignment of gaze serving as a prefatory package to the production or continuation of the activity. The speaker employs movement to gain the recipient's attention to and involvement in the utterance, the business, or the topic at hand.

The elicitation of gaze through body movement may stand in other relations with the surrounding talk. For example in Fragment 3:4 the foot movement which successfully encourages Jennifer to look up is preceded and accompanied by other, vocal attempts to elicit a response from the candidate recipient. The foot movement, accompanied by the second "Jennifer" is used following the failure of "which Jennifer" to gain a response; it is as if the visual action is a tougher attempt, an upgraded device, to gain the recipient's attention. Similarly in Fragment 3:6 the patient's leg cross follows pauses and other disfluencies within the articulation of the utterance which themselves may well be attempts to encourage the doctor to shift the focus of his attention. In both cases a movement appears to be used following the failure of other devices embedded in the talk to elicit the gaze of the cointeractant. In these examples it is as if body movement is employed where other devices have failed, increasing the pressure on the other to respond.

However, attempts to encourage another to realign his gaze through body movement are not always used following the failure of previous attempts produced in the talk. In Fragment 3:1 for example the speaker begins by tugging at Lythia's shoulder, and on the failure of the initial movements to elicit a response follows with a wave. Similarly in Fragments 3:2, 3:3, and 3:5 the attempts to elicit the recipient's gaze through nonvocal action do not follow earlier attempts through disfluency in speech. There appears to be no general rule or procedure to explain why movement is used rather than other devices to encourage recipient activity. Encouraging another to realign his gaze through movement may occur alone or in juxtaposition to other devices. It is used both when the potential recipient is simply looking away and when he is engaged in an alternative activity such as reading the medical records. And surprisingly in the face of other studies (Beattie 1978a, 1979, 1983; C. Goodwin 1979a, 1980, 1981a; Kendon 1967), its use and position in or with an utterance appears to bear no systematic relation to the gaze direction of the speaker. It would seem that speakers have available a range of devices for realigning another's gaze or more generally encouraging recipient activity, and which device they actually employ turns on the activity in which they are engaged and the circumstances at hand. For example gesture and the like can be used to distinguish fellow participants.

Differentiating recipient participation and selecting next speaker

Unlike many of the examples, Fragments 3:1 and 3:4 are drawn from interviews which involve more than two participants. In such circumstances one issue that arises is whether the speaker is attempting to gain the attention of all those co-present, or differentiating the participants in some fashion. Both fragments appear to involve some form of recipient selection. In Fragment 3:4 the leg tap and the vocal summons unambiguously select Jennifer as the primary recipient, and the utterance itself is coordinated with her nonvocal behaviour, the shift of gaze to the speaker. The interviewer does not exclude the mother as a listener, but rather differentiates the obligations the cointeractants have towards the activity. Superficially Fragment 3:1 looks rather similar; the speaker's gestures encourage a particular participant to respond, with Lythia during the utterance briefly turning towards her father and displaying at least minimal participation. Recall, however, that it is actually the doctor who replies, and though the utterance is apparently addressed to Lythia it is in fact the doctor more than any other participant who might have something to say on the subject of his two daughters. The father's utterance, whilst not interrupting the activity of writing the prescription, perhaps indirectly encourages the doctor to participate whilst avoiding speaking directly to him or selecting him as next speaker. The utterance and its accompanying gesture serve to differentiate the obligations that others have towards the activity and how they should participate in it. Lythia is encouraged to display receipt in its course and the doctor is perhaps encouraged to reply on its completion.[6]

In the following fragment a movement is used to establish a person as a recipient and thereby select her as next speaker. The example is drawn from the same interview as Fragment 3:4, as the social worker is discovering the difficulties entailed in encouraging Jennifer to participate.

Fragment 3:7 Transcript 1

```
SW:   do you feel thats a fair comment? about you
      (.5)
SW:   I'm sorry I didn't getchur:: (.)first name
J:    =⎡⎡Jennifer
M:     ⎣⎣Jennifer
SW:   hhhuh heh do:you feel thats fair::
      (1.0)
E:    hmᵒdon't know
```

Following a diatribe by the mother concerning how the teachers find Jennifer at school, the interviewer turns to her client and asks her opinion. Jennifer is staring at the floor and produces neither vocal nor visual response. Following an intervening sequence of talk,[7] the question is recycled by the social worker and successfully elicits a somewhat minimal reply from Jennifer. In the intervening sequence the interviewer not only establishes Jennifer as a recipient but also as a speaker, a fully fledged participant, if only temporarily, in the interaction.

Fragment 3:7 Transcript 2

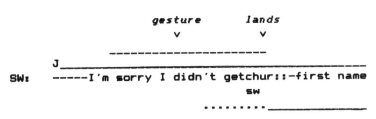

```
            gesture       lands
              v             v
      ----------------------------
   J_____
SW:   -----I'm sorry I didn't getchur::-first name
                          sw
              . . . . . . . . ._____
```

On receiving no reply to her initial question the interviewer asks Jennifer's name. With her question is coupled a gesture. The social worker reaches forward and squeezes Jennifer's knee, withdrawing the hand prior to the completion of her utterance. As the hand travels towards its target Jennifer looks up, turning from the floor to the social worker. In eliciting the client's gaze the social worker establishes her as the recipient of the utterance, an utterance which obliges Jennifer to speak following its completion. In integrating Jennifer into the interaction as an active participant, the interviewer follows her reply with a next question, a recycled version of the inquiry concerning how Jennifer felt about the teachers' comments. The social worker returns to the business at hand and in so doing captures Jennifer as a recipient, a recipient of a question of which she cannot pretend ignorance. Jennifer utters "hm°don't know" and returns her gaze to the floor. The package of actions between the two questions establishes Jennifer's involvement in the business at hand as both a recipient and speaker.

The nonvocal action of a speaker therefore can be used to differentiate those present and encourage certain forms of participation from particular persons. An accompanying body movement can serve to locate a particular interactant as the primary recipient of an utterance and to display publicly to others within the perceptual range of the activity how they should behave towards both the speaker and the selected party. Moreover the package of utterance and movement can be fashioned in such a way as to encourage, directly and indirectly, certain forms of response from particular persons. And in differentiating recipients, speakers can establish a particular person as the relevent next speaker. In using movements to differentiate how persons behave during the utterance, a speaker thereby implicates how the activity should be dealt with following its completion.

Sustaining multiparty participation

It has been seen how a movement such as a gesture might be used to differentiate cointeractants and establish a particular person as the primary recipient of an activity. In the following fragment gestures are used to elicit a response from all those present and to encourage continuing involvement in the activity at hand. The fragment captures a long and complex stretch of interaction. For both economy and clarity it will be best to select a few extracts and discuss them in detail.

Fragment 3:8   Transcript 1

```
Dr:    and this is a very common complaint to people
       who've had this operation done
       (.)
H:     Oh::: (.2) well that makes me a lot happier
       (.3)
H:     you ⌈know I was getting eh bit wer::(.)well my wife
W:        ⌊hhhhhhhhhhhhhhhh
H:     was getting a bit concerned becos now it's gone
       milder today
       (.)
Dr:    yes
H:     just the difference
       (.4)
H:     but I'm a bit concerned about taking panadols or
       something like that what would you suggestse:tthhh
       do ah need to take anything for ⌈this
Dr:                                     ⌊not if
       the pain isn't severe (.2) erm: ⌈:
H:                                      ⌊no: : I ⌈haven't
W:                                              ⌊well it..
```

The consultation involves three participants, a husband and wife, both
of whom are patients, and the doctor. The husband presents his problem
first; the fragment begins as the doctor mentions it is a very common
complaint. The husband voices his pleasure and over successive utterances elaborates his concerns. As the patient begins to voice his happiness
he is faced with potential recipients who are looking elsewhere. His wife
is looking at the doctor and the doctor to one side with his eyes closed.
Following "Oh:::" the speaker begins a gesture. In a broad circumference
he sweeps his right hand past his wife and projects it towards the doctor.
As the hand passes his wife she turns and looks at her husband; as it
nears the doctor he opens his eyes and looks at the speaker. In the course
of the utterance the speaker successfully encourages both cointeractants
to realign their gaze and display their involvement in the activity at hand.
A single gesture accomplishes this work; it establishes multiple participation in the utterance.

Fragment 3:8   Drawings 1 and 2

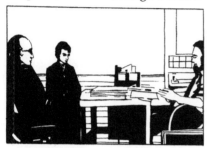 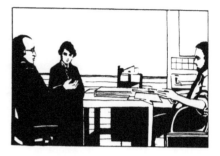

```
       D1                      D2.
H:   Oh:::--well that makes me a lot happier
```

By the end of the utterance in which he attributes concern to his wife, the patient no longer has the gaze of either cointeractant. He produces "becos," projecting more to follow, and then pauses. With the word "becos" the speaker lifts his hand and slices the air. As it begins to slice, it catches the eye of his fellow interactants; the doctor and wife both turn towards the speaker. As their gaze arrives the husband continues his utterance, giving an example of the variability of the complaint.

Fragment 3:8   Transcript 2

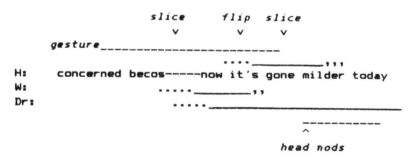

This is different from the first example, however, in that the speaker continues to gesture following the receipt of the cointeractants' gaze. After slicing the air he flips the hand to one side, nearest his wife, and as if in response she turns away from the speaker. Once more the speaker begins to slice the air and in harmony the doctor rocks his head up and down, as if agreeing with the utterance. The continuing gesture serves to attract a show of heightened involvement in the activity at hand from one of its recipients.

Fragment 3:8 Transcript 3

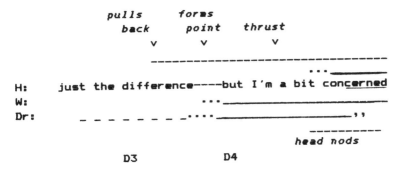

```
                pulls       forms
                 back       point    thrust
                  v          v         v

                ------------------------------------
                                       ..._____
H:     just the difference----but I'm a bit concerned
W:                            ..._____
Dr:        _ _ _ _ _ _ _._...._____''
                                       ----------
                                       head nods
           D3                 D4
```

With "just the difference" the speaker brings to an end his example of the way in which cold weather can affect his complaint. The wife is looking at the doctor, and the doctor turns and begins to read the medical record cards. Far from finishing the discussion concerning his illness, the husband displays his desire to continue. As he brings his utterance to an end, with "difference" he begins a gesture, thrusting his hand towards his own knee. He then raises his hand, drawing it back towards his face. As the hand moves, the doctor turns from the records to the face of the speaker. The hand travels towards the speaker's face and whilst passing the wife begins to form a point, a point which is thrust at his own nose. In forming a point, the gesture attracts the gaze of the wife, and she turns to the potential speaker. The movement serves to encourage both cointeractants to turn and display attention to the potential speaker. On beginning the utterance the speaker is secure in the light of receiving a demonstration that both the doctor and the wife are prepared to participate in the upcoming activity. And to cap it all, as the speaker points at his own face he moves the point back and forth, and the doctor starts to nod his head in synchrony.

Fragment 3:8 Drawings 3 and 4

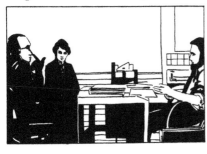
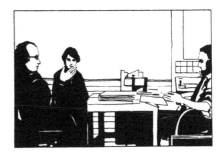

Whereas in earlier examples it was found that speakers could employ body movement to differentiate the obligations that particular interactants have towards an utterance, in Fragment 3:8 the speaker uses a single movement to realign the gaze of both cointeractants and establish their involvement in the activity at hand. And in a couple of instances the speaker coordinates the articulation of the utterance with the visual behaviour of both the doctor and his wife, withholding talk until both potential recipients have displayed their preparedness to participate in the activity. The stretch of interaction seems almost akin to a lecture or speech in which one party attempts to maintain the involvement of an audience through a succession of interrelated utterances. The speaker's broad sweeping gestures, flamboyant enough to elicit smiles from a next-of-kin, appear designed to elicit the gaze of all those present rather than select a particular recipient. However ornate, the husband's gestural activity meets with some success. Not only does the husband hold the floor and continue to talk across a series of turns, prolonging the discussion of his common complaint, but in so doing maintains the continuing participation and involvement of both cointeractants in the details of his troubles.

Having said this, it remains clear that though the speaker's gestures serve to liven both members of the audience, it is the doctor rather than the wife who is the primary recipient. It is the doctor who is unfamiliar with the patient's woes and who may have to proffer appreciation and advice on the complaint. Moreover, though the speaker's gestures serve to encourage participation from both cointeractants, it is the doctor to whom they are specifically addressed. The gestures sweep past the wife and perform their work in front of the doctor. It is there that they serve to encourage further activity from their main recipient, successive head nods in time with the hand's movement, a show of heightened participation in the husband's concerns. However, though the doctor is the primary recipient and has particular obligations towards the speaker, the wife through her sensitivity to the nonvocal actions of her husband displays her continued attention to his talk. By coordinating her visual alignment with her husband's gestures, the wife demonstrates her involvement in and perhaps appreciation of his complaint and its details. Simply by withholding responses to a speaker's gestures through a stretch of talk primarily between two cointeractants, a third party can avoid such alignment and accomplish very different sorts of work. And, as we are all aware, such actions between husband and wife are not insignificant and can give rise to severe difficulties in that long drive home after the event.

Discussion: the interactional design of body movement

In the preceding chapter it was suggested that pause could be used to elicit another's gaze. A speaker can withhold a sequentially appropriate next utterance or pause within the course of a turn and thereby encourage a cointeractant to realign his visual orientation. In this chapter we have found that body movement may also be used to elicit gaze, the first movement projecting a sequentially relevant next action in a particular position. The tight sequential ordering of the two-action sequence provides interactants with the possibility of inspecting what occurs immediately following the first action in order to discern whether the appropriate response has occurred. And, as has been seen in Fragment 3:1 and elsewhere, on finding the relevant action absent, further attempts, frequently through modified or new gestures, are used to elicit the appropriate response.

The elicitation of gaze through body movement can stand independently, as a device for example which serves to initiate an encounter such as occurs when one hails a taxi and it draws to the kerb. It also takes place in face-to-face interaction both with and within talk. For example a speaker in the course of an utterance may use a gesture or some other form of movement to elicit a response from a candidate recipient; the nonvocal actions of both participants occur alongside the talk, the speaker gathering the recipient in its course. In other instances the utterance or part of the utterance is withheld until the speaker has successfully elicited the gaze of the cointeractant, the production of the utterance being interactionally coordinated through the visual and vocal behaviour of the participants. It is also found that the elicitation of gaze through body movement may be coordinated with disfluencies that occur within the utterance itself. The gestural attempt to elicit gaze may follow previous attempts produced through perturbations in the talk. Thus in articulating an utterance the speaker is sensitive to the behaviour of the recipient and employs nonvocal action to secure the attention of the cointeractant(s).

Speakers in face-to-face interaction do not of course necessarily require the gaze of a recipient;[8] many utterances occur with no apparent difficulty without the speaker securing or attempting to secure a cointeractant's gaze. Should, however, a speaker wish to receive the gaze of another or encourage other forms of participation from a cointeractant, then gestural activity and other types of movement can be employed to fashion the responsibilities that a recipient(s) has towards an utterance(s). The movement sets the way in which the cointeractant should receive the activity of the speaker. It operates locally, utterance by utterance, frequently displaying in the course of speaking how the cointeractant should behave towards the activity. These movements to encourage a realignment of gaze by the recipient may be used in a variety of positions within an utterance. Some occur at utterance beginning, others deep into the utterance itself. They can be used to encourage involvement wherever the speaker should so wish,[9] perhaps for an utterance or successive utterances, perhaps for a couple of crucial words within a stretch of talk.

Some of the examples of movement eliciting gaze have the flavour of the prefatory package mentioned in Chapter 2; others do not. Unlike pauses, restarts, and other speech disfluencies that may serve to encourage recipient activity, encouraging another to realign his gaze through gesture and the like does not necessarily delay the utterance. As shown, it can occur alongside the utterance, gathering an audience in its course. For the speaker, however, this does run the risk of completing the utterance without eliciting the other's gaze and possibly undermining the sequential force of the activity. In other instances the speaker withholds talk until he successfully encourages the other to realign gaze. The movement and the reorientation of gaze serve as a package that sets the appropriate scene prior to the articulation or continuation of an activity. The activity is then produced in the light of an environment that entails a cointeractant displaying preparedness to participate in and attend to the speaker's actions.

A disparate collection of physical movements are used to elicit another's gaze. Even in the small collection of examples discussed here we find posture shifts, leg taps, and various forms of gesture. These different forms of physical movement are all used to perform a similar type of social action: to encourage another to display recipiency to the activities of a speaker. If one considers the various circumstances in which the actions are produced it soon becomes apparent that no single physical movement could successfully elicit another's gaze on each and every occasion. For example the graduate's posture shift in Fragment 3:2 could well have passed unnoticed by Jennifer, and it would be inappropriate as well as difficult for Mr. Arman to tap the doctor's leg. In various ways the different movements used to encourage another to realign his or her gaze pertain to the circumstances at hand and the contingencies faced by the speaker; they are designed to accomplish a given action at a particular moment in the course of the interaction.

As many studies demonstrate (including Birdwhistell 1970; Condon and Ogston 1966, 1967, 1971; Kendon 1977; Scheflen 1973), face-to-face interaction involves a continual flow of mutually coordinated body movement, ranging from eye and facial behaviour to major shifts in orientation. Within this continual flow of nonvocal behaviour, relatively few movements serve to attract the gaze of the cointeractants. The movements which do elicit another's gaze stand out from the surrounding and co-occurring behaviour; they render themselves noticeable and serve to catch the eye of one or more of the persons co-present. In some fashion the movements contrast with the local environment of goings-on; they protrude within the local milieu and thereby alter the other's visual orientation. In standing out, the movements enter the foreground and reflexively set co-occurring movements into the background. The local scene is momentarily recast.

It has been suggested by Hall (1963, 1966, 1968), Sommer (1959), Sommer and Becker (1974), and a number of other researchers that in face-to-face interaction the spatial arrangements of particular categories of individual remain relatively stable. One way in which the movements used to elicit another's gaze stand out in the local environment is by temporarily altering the spatial arrangement. For example in Fragment 3:7 the psychiatric social worker moves towards Jennifer and places her hand on the knee; in Fragment 3:2 the speaker shifts posturally towards the candidate recipient; and in Fragment 3:1 the speaker waves his hand by the side of his daughter's face. In these and many other cases, the speaker projects part of his body closer to the co-interactant, closing up the distance between the participants and entering the territorial surrounds of the other. Even in Fragment 3:6, one of the few examples where the speaker moves posturally away from his potential recipient, it is worth noting that in crossing his legs his knee travels upward towards the doctor.

In temporarily altering the spatial arrangements between the interactants, the movement which serves to elicit another's gaze frequently projects a body part towards the other's line of regard. Consider for example the leg tap or knee grab used by the psychiatric social worker. Both movements reach into the area between the client's face and the floor; both cross the focus of her visual orientation. Or consider the way in which in leaning sideways towards the doctor in Fragment 3:2 the patient brings himself close to the area of the recipient's activity and the focus of his attention. And in examples such as Fragments 3:1 and 3:5 where the first attempt to elicit the other's gaze through movement fails, the second or third attempt entails moving part of the body still closer to the candidate recipient's field of vision. In Fragment 3:5 for instance, the circling gesture makes a successively broader circumference and finally thrusts close to the doctor's domain of activity. The gesture is modified in the course of its articulation, progressively moving part of the body closer to the doctor's line of regard so as to achieve the particular task to which it is addressed.

However, the movements do not necessarily have to cross the other's line of regard to draw the other's gaze; rather they appear to operate on the periphery of the visual field. As students of cognition and eye movement have demonstrated – for example Friedman and Liebelt 1981; Maurer and Lewis 1981; Stark and Ellis 1981 – human beings are extremely sensitive to sudden changes outside the direct line of their regard and on the perimeter of their vision. By projecting a body part to the periphery rather than directly across the recipient's line of regard, a speaker can simply indicate that something is happening and catch another's eye. In this way he may encourage the other to realign his attention, rather than demand it – not unlike knocking on a door rather than walking straight in.[10] The movements respect the momentary concerns and territorial rights of the other; they operate in the wings, trading on our ability to notice changes on the margins of our attention. And it is interesting to observe that the more gross movements, the demands rather than requests for another's attention, not infrequently follow earlier and gentler attempts to encourage the cointeractant to attend. Finding the other failing to respond to hints rather than demands on his attention, a speaker increases the pressure on the other to realign his gaze, moving part of his body progressively closer to and sometimes invading the recipient's line of regard.

Condon and Ogston (1966, 1967, 1971), Kendon (1977), Scheflen (1973), more recently Erickson and Schultz (1982) and Kempton (1980), and other students of visual behaviour have demonstrated how human beings in interaction develop stable, mutually coordinated rhythms of body movement. As well as altering the spatial arrangements of the individuals, movements which serve to encourage another to realign his gaze often alter the rhythmical structure of behavioural coordination, momentarily shifting the pace of the interaction. In Fragment 3:8 for example the withdrawal of the speaker's hand to his own face is a sudden and accentuated movement, momentarily accelerating the pace in contrast to the slow projection forward a moment earlier. In Fragment 3:3 the stomach clutch by the speaker stands out from the gentle flow of movement, and in Fragment 3:5 the patient's gesture thrusts towards the recipient, breaking the pace of the movement up until that moment. The movements break with the environment of activity; they disjunct the interaction and produce a temporary dissynchrony in the interactional rhythm.[11] These observations reflect recent research by Erickson and

Schultz (1982) concerned with the counselling interview, in which they show how difficulties in communication are reflected in dissynchrony between the participants in their speech and body movement. In the instances discussed here of course, movement that stands out from the local environment of activity is being used to solve interactional difficulties concerning the attention of the participants to the business at hand.

In the foregoing, the exotic and extraordinary nature of movements designed to realign another's gaze has been mentioned. It has been suggested that such movements stand out from the environment of goings-on to catch another's eye, that they momentarily alter the spatial arrangements of the individuals and shift the rhythmical structure of behaviour. Yet the movements in question are very ordinary – postural shifts, gestures, leg taps; little of the remarkable or the dramatic. If, however, the sole concern of such movements was to attract the attention of another, then one might well expect to find more theatrical manoeuvres. A person would have little difficulty in attracting the attention of the other if he were to thump the desk, thrust his hands in front of another's eyes, or whip the medical records from under his nose. In adult interaction, and certainly in the medical consultation, such flamboyant moves to attract another's attention are rare.

In each example it is the speaker or potential speaker who uses movement to realign the gaze of the cointeractant(s). In eliciting another's gaze the speaker is attempting to encourage the potential recipient to attend to an utterance or utterances. The gesture, postural shift, or whatever works on behalf of the activity with which it occurs; its task is to establish a recipient for the utterance. The movement is the servant of the talk; it works to secure a recipient, to have the activity attended to and thereby accomplish its sequential relevance and interactional force. The more theatrical or forceful a movement, the more it risks drawing the other's eyes to itself rather than to the face of the speaker. An extraordinary movement, though succeeding in eliciting another's gaze, might well be noticed and attended to in its own right, perhaps even lead to question and complaint. In thrusting itself into the limelight, the movement would fail to gain attention for the talk it accompanies; it would serve itself rather than its master. Thus more theatrical or forceful movements[12] might well undermine the very action they were set to achieve; they would direct attention elsewhere rather than assist the sequential relevance or performative force of the utterance they accompany. The movement is designed primarily to establish and maintain involvement in the accompanying talk, the business or topic at hand. It serves to align the co-participant's attention to something other than itself, the talk with which it occurs. Hence it is hardly surprising that so many operate on the periphery. There they can catch another's eye without drawing attention to themselves.

As a social organization, the elicitation of gaze through body movement is flexible; it occurs in a variety of interactional locations and informs the maintenance of involvement in a broad range of interactional settings. It is used to establish another's attention or can serve to differentiate potential recipients, beckoning the participation of a particular party and excluding others. In large gatherings such as lectures, public talks, even auctions, we can observe how gestural activity can serve to maintain the attention of an audience. It is also interesting to observe how more specialized forms of communication trade on the ability of sudden and contrasting movements to draw the attention of human beings. Television commercials for example not infrequently gain the viewer's attention by repeated shifts in visual presentation, and in poster campaigns we find advertisers simulating movement in still pictures in an attempt to catch a person's eye. Consider for example the poster below drawn from a campaign by International Distillers and Vintners to publicize a brand of gin. There is evidence to suggest that the poster was successful in attracting people's gazes, though perhaps it came too close to shifting people's attention to the method rather than the message.

The ability to elicit the gaze of others through visual action provides a systematic solution to the issue so acutely raised by Goffman (1967).

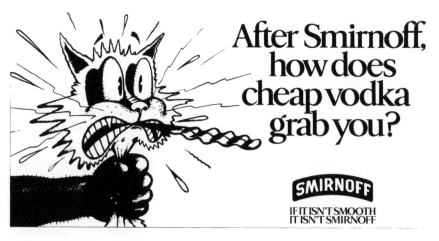

Poster advertisement.

People can use body movement to encourage each other to attend and participate in an activity, the business at hand, without addressing the problem of involvement as a topic in its own right. Movement establishes the involvement of others, their integration in an action or activity, yet masks its own operations; it is a device whose very success rests on its invisibility.

4. Forms of participation

"Participation framework." When a word is spoken, all those
who happen to be in perceptual range of the event will have
some sort of participation status relative to it. The codification of
these various positions and the normative specification of
appropriate conduct within each provide an essential
background for interaction analysis–whether (I presume) in our
own society or any other.

Goffman 1981, p. 3

A change in footing implies a change in the alignment we take
up to ourselves and the others present as expressed in the way
we manage the production or reception of an utterance. A
change in our footing is another way of talking about a change
in our frame of events. . . . Participants over the course of their
speaking constantly change their footing, these changes being a
persistent feature of natural talk.

Ibid., p. 128

The method consists of treating an actual appearance as "the
document of," as "pointing to," as "standing on behalf of" a
pre-supposed underlying pattern. Not only is the underlying
pattern derived from its individual documentary evidences, but
the individual documentary evidences, in their turn, are
interpreted on the basis of "what is known" about the
underlying pattern. Each is used to elaborate the other.

Garfinkel 1967, p. 78

In previous chapters it has been suggested that by turning towards the
face of another a person may display his or her willingness to receive
an action or activity. So for example it is found that during the course
of an utterance a speaker may withhold talk until the potential recipient
has turned his gaze and thereby displayed attention to the actions of
the speaker. In encouraging another to turn towards his face through
gesture and the like, a speaker is not concerned with having a co-par-

ticipant inspect his face but rather show attention to the utterance. The co-participant almost has to look at the speaker but not see him, in a sense to look through the speaker to the activity in which he is engaged. There are, however, occasions where a person may not simply desire to have another turn towards his face but rather to take notice of a phenomenon in the local milieu. It may be a piece of furniture, a gesture, or a passing friend; an object, an activity, or a person. In pointing out or showing something or someone to another, the participant is invited to realign his visual orientation and refocus his attention, taking note of a particular phenomenon that might otherwise pass unseen. In pointing out or showing an object to another an interactant can topicalize a feature within the local environment and render it relevant to an activity and the business at hand.

In some cases successfully encouraging someone to notice a phenomenon in the local environment can constitute a distinct episode in itself. For example showing another he has dropped his handkerchief and then picking it up may terminate, perhaps to the regret of both participants, a brief encounter. Or for instance in Fragment 1:1 we saw the way a child might point out the camera to her parent whilst the doctor is engaged elsewhere, the episode ending as the participants chuckle and return their attention to the medical practitioner. Yet not infrequently pointing and showing occur within the topic at hand and serve to temporarily realign the visual attention of the interactants as they talk and deal with particular contingencies which may arise.

The medical consultation abounds with examples of persons pointing out and showing objects and the like to each other. Outside the formal physical examination, patients in the course of disclosing their troubles frequently invite doctors to inspect the surface manifestations of their complaints—spots on the hand, a bruised leg, or a twisted knee. In such cases, patients render themselves the focus of involvement, no longer to be looked at and not seen, but rather to become the object of visual attention and inspection. These pointings and showings frequently occur as the patient talks to the doctor and consequently necessitate a shift in the sorts of responsibilities and obligations that the recipient has towards the speaker and the activity.

Revealing an object in the course of speaking

In the course of talking, a speaker may encourage a recipient to look at and take notice of an object in the local environment.[1]

Fragment 4:1 Transcript 1

```
P:      I got something come up on my back < it started
        like little white
        (.2)
P:      blotches
Dr:     yeah
P:      and it's now spread an spread an spread
        (.5)
P:      I've had crea:ms: and everything(.)<an it wont
        (.7)
P:      go
        (.8)
Dr:     oh:: yes:
        (.2)
P:      it's now going across my shou:lders an::(.)it(.)
        <I never worried about it until somebody said euee
        :::::::: whats all that
```

Even before the beginning of this fragment, the patient, unrequested by the doctor, has begun to undress. By "it's now spread" the patient has unbuttoned his shirt and is standing facing the doctor. As the patient speaks he holds a face-to-face orientation with the doctor, the doctor gazes at the patient's face and takes no apparent notice of the patient being partially undressed and the naked stomach protruding towards him. Following the doctor's "oh:: yes:" the patient continues the description of his symptoms, with the doctor no longer gazing at his face but inspecting his back.

Fragment 4:1   Drawings 1 and 2

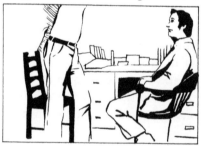 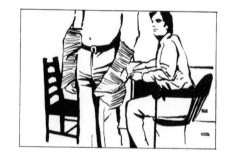

Towards the completion of the first part of the description of his complaint, the patient encourages the doctor to realign his gaze. At "won't" the patient shifts gaze away from the doctor and turns round, showing his back to the doctor. As the patient begins to turn round, the doctor stands to take a closer look at the complaint. On looking at the back the doctor utters "oh:: yes:," and the patient continues the description of the trouble.

Fragment 4:1 Transcript 2

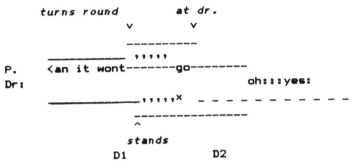

In pausing and turning round, the patient invites the doctor temporarily to suspend his face-to-face orientation with the cointeractant and visually inspect the back. Showing the back places the recipient under certain obligations; it locates an interactional position where the recipient should rearrange the fashion in which he is participating in the activities of the speaker. The patient withholds showing his back almost until the completion of the turn at talk and the first part of the description. He maintains the face-to-face orientation during the description and as it draws to a close sets the activity in motion, the realignment of the recipient's gaze occurring at the completion of the utterance and serving as a junction between the initial description and its continued elaboration.

A speaker may realign the recipient's gaze earlier in an utterance and use that realignment as a way of completing a particular activity.

Fragment 4:2 Transcript 1

```
P:      an once I looked(.)<I don't whether (it's a)
        connected or not
        (.8)
P:      but I've got a big bruise on my leg
        (.5)
P:      an it looks:
        (.7)
P:      (0 just there)
        (.7)
P:      it was sore yes:terday
        (.4)
P:      its: not
        (1.0)
P:      so bad today
Dr:     did you hur:t yourself there as well when
        you:: (.)hurt your ankle
```

As with Fragment 4:1, we enter the consultation as the patient describes her complaint. She identifies the difficulty as "big bruise on my leg" and goes on to suggest that she will describe the appearance of the problem. The projected description introduced by "an it looks:" is vocally unforthcoming, and a second or so later the patient continues by mentioning that the complaint is less severe today than yesterday. Throughout the fragment, up until the gap following "an it looks:," the speaker and recipient are in a face-to-face orientation, the recipient gazing at the speaker during the naming of the problem and the following vocalization. By the time the patient continues with "it was sore" both doctor and patient are looking at the object in question, the bruise on the leg.

Fragment 4:2   Drawings 1 and 2

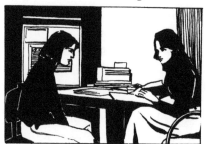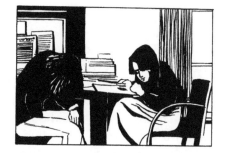

The doctor's gaze arrives at the patient's leg approximately 0.5 second into the gap following "looks:." The shift in orientation from the patient's face to her leg occurs in juxtaposition to particular nonvocal actions by the speaker. In pausing, the speaker turns from the recipient to the knee and simultaneously drops her hands and lifts her trouser leg. As the speaker's gaze shifts and her hands drop towards her leg, the recipient turns towards the object; "(°just there)" is coordinated with the doctor's gaze arriving at the leg and entails the patient fixing the precise point with her finger.

Fragment 4:2 Transcript 2

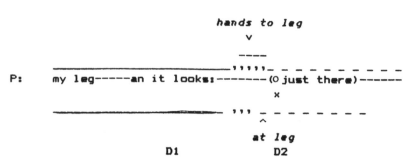

In the course of the utterance or projected utterance, the speaker through her nonvocal actions invites the recipient to realign her gaze, to turn from the speaker's face to the leg. The speaker's nonvocal actions encourage the recipient to alter the ways in which she participates in the activity at hand, from orientating towards the speaker face to face to inspecting an object in the local environment. And in gaining the recipient's cooperation in turning towards the object, it is no longer incumbent on the speaker to complete the vocal description of the bruise on the leg. The activity of describing the appearance of the difficulty is accomplished by the co-participant actually viewing the object in question. The patient produces the activity both vocally and visually, redesigning the articulation of the activity in its course. She succeeds in this form of production by successfully encouraging the doctor to alter the way in which she participates in the activity at hand.

The participants' realignment towards the leg follows an earlier attempt where the patient is unsuccessful in encouraging the doctor to look at the object. During "but I've got" the patient turns from the doctor to the leg and drops her hands to her trousers in a fashion not dissimilar to the later example. The doctor remains orientated towards the speaker, gazing at her face, and by "big bruise" the patient has returned her gaze once more to the doctor. Consequently it is found, as the vocalization "(°just there)" also suggests, that in attempting to realign the orientation of the recipient, the speaker is sensitive to how the recipient responds to the invitation and is able to undertake remedial action so as not to produce an activity which is lacking the appropriate form of co-participation. The second attempt is produced in the light of the first; not only does it reproduce similar nonvocal action, but simultaneously the projected description is withheld, stalling the activity's progress.

Thus in both instances the speaker during an utterance successfully realigns the gaze of the recipient and renders an object noticeable. In the first instance the speaker shows the object to his fellow participant; in the second the speaker points the object out to the recipient. The realignment of the recipient's gaze is locally coordinated with the shift in orientation by the speaker and perhaps the accompanying pause. Just as a pause may serve to elicit a recipient's gaze to the face of the speaker, so it may encourage other forms of recipient activity.[2] In the cases described here, the speaker prior to pausing has the gaze of the recipient, a necessity if one is going to point out or reveal a particular object to another person. The speaker's nonvocal actions coupled with the pause serve to encourage the recipient to realign his or her gaze and focus on the object invited by the speaker.

Showing or pointing out an object in the course of an utterance and a stretch of talk encourages the recipient to change his behaviour towards the speaker. The relevance of a face-to-face orientation is temporarily lifted. The speaker in inviting the recipient to look elsewhere proposes an alternative set of obligations, a proper way of behaving towards the speaker and the activity at hand. In shifting the way in which he is producing the activity from vocally describing the complaint to actually showing it, the speaker requires the cooperation of the recipient, not only to listen and display he is listening, but to inspect visually an object in the local environment.

Establishing a visual framework at utterance beginning

In some cases an interactant may encourage another to look at an object in the local milieu at the beginning of an utterance.

Fragment 4:3   Transcript 1

```
Dr:    What bringesth you this morning
       (.6)
P:     er::m:(.)I've got these::(.)aw:ful spots:
       (.5)
Dr:    (oh::) ⌈yes
P:            ⌊on my fin:gers:
       (1.2)
P:     been there for a long time actually<I've been
       about them before
```

As the doctor asks what brought the patient he reads the medical record cards. By the end of "er::m:," actually before the patient has begun the utterance proper, the doctor has not only turned around but focused on the object of the patient's complaint, spots on her fingers. From then on, throughout the whole fragment the doctor looks at the patient's fingers and never towards her face.

Fragment 4:3   Transcript 2

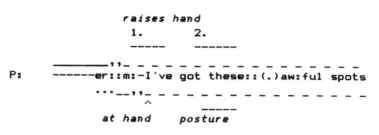

```
                    raises hand
                    1.        2.
                    -----     ------

         ————————,,_ _ _ _ _ _ _ _ _ _ _ _ _ _ _ _
P:       ------er::m:-I've got these::(.)aw:ful spots
         ···_—,,_ _ _ _ _ _ _ _ _ _ _ _ _ _ _ _
                    ^
         at hand    posture
```

Following a 0.6-second gap the patient begins her reply, producing "er::m:" and then pausing. The "er::m:" appears to elicit the gaze of the doctor, and he turns from the medical record cards to the patient's face.[3] As she utters "er::m:" the patient turns from the doctor to her own hand and simultaneously raises her hand towards her potential recipient. In turning towards her hand the patient raises her eyebrows and opens her eyes wide, exaggerating her looking at the object. Consequently as the doctor turns round to face the patient he finds her neither gazing towards him nor simply looking away but rather looking at something. He immediately turns and detects the object in question, the patient's spots. She pauses following "er::m:," only continuing with the content of the utterance as the doctor's gaze arrives at her hand.

The patient not only elicits the gaze of the recipient prior to beginning the content of the utterance but successfully encourages the cointeractant to look at her hand. Even prior to identifying her problem vocally, the patient has encouraged the doctor to observe the complaint. And as he looks at the object she raises it closer to his eyes, allowing him a more detailed inspection of the as yet unmentioned "aw:ful spots:." As he turns round, the doctor uses the direction of the speaker's gaze and the raising hand to determine where he should look, what he should look at, and how he should participate in the activity, the patient's vocal and visual actions.

The following instance is rather similar.

Fragment 4:4   Transcript 1

```
Dr:   Wha::t can we do for you Mister Howard
P:    Err::(.)it's:: this: doctor:er::
      (.2)
Dr:   Errerr thats a ⌈good specimen<when did it come up
P:                   ⌊err
P:    Err::(.)well its::(.)been coming over the:(.)weekend
      like you know
           yes
```

Again it is drawn from the beginning of a consultation where the doctor is ignorant of the patient's reason for the visit. During the initial question the doctor turns from the patient to the medical record cards. By the word "this:" during the patient's reply the doctor has turned from the records and is moving to take a closer look at the patient's eye, the source of his trouble.

Fragment 4:4   Transcript 2

```
         point
           v

         --------
     -----------,,,,,
P:              Err::(.)it's:: this: doctor:er::
Dr:      Howard

           ,,,,, _ _ _ _ _ _ _ _ _ _ _ _ _
           ----------
               ^
         moves closer
```

The shift of gaze by the doctor from the records to the patient's face
appears responsive to the gesture which accompanies the "err::" at the
beginning of the utterance. In turning towards the face of the patient,
the doctor finds the speaker pointing to his own eye and moving his
face closer to the recipient. The doctor moves closer to inspect the eye
and as he does the patient begins the content of the utterance with "it's::
this: doctor:er::." As in Fragment 4:3, the speaker elicits the cointeractant's gaze to the face and then encourages the recipient to look at a
particular object. Meanwhile the content of the utterance is withheld
until the recipient aligns his gaze towards the object.[4]

As in the examples discussed earlier, in Fragments 4:3 and 4:4 the
speaker encourages the recipient to look at and take notice of an object
in the local milieu. In these instances the speaker from the start of the
utterance attempts to realign the obligations that the cointeractant has
as a recipient. The speaker invites the potential recipient to temporarily
suspend a face-to-face orientation and establish the object in question
as the focus of visual attention. The speaker encourages the cointeractant
to participate in a certain fashion and on receiving the cooperation of
the other successfully establishes a certain framework of participation
for the utterance and its accompanying visual action. The framework
allows the activity to be produced and understood in a certain way.

In both instances the patient's activities are responsive to an utterance
in which the doctor initiates the business of the consultation. The appointments are both new visits by the patient where the doctor is initially
ignorant of the patient's reason for the call. In responding to the doctor
the patient collaborates in starting the business at hand and begins by
providing the reason for the visit. In realigning the gaze of the doctor
to the object the patient encourages the potential recipient to participate
in the activity in a particular fashion. In securing the doctor's cooperation
the interactants establish a certain participation framework, a specific

form of producing the activity and having it attended to, a form which allows the patient to show the complaint rather than merely describe it. In securing the doctor as an active viewer as well as a hearer the patient can allow his description to inform the actual appearance of the complaint and the actual appearance to elaborate the description, vocal and visual being thoroughly interrelated in the activity's articulation. Moreover the participation framework initiated by the patient informs how the activity is accomplished through a consecutive series of utterances.

Withholding talk for a noticing

In some cases a person may withhold an activity until he has received an appropriate orientation from a recipient.

Fragment 4:5 Transcript 1

```
Dr:     All right
        (.)
Dr:     put them back on
P:      Well
Dr:     < w┌ell:
P:        └ see that one
        (1.4)
P:      I was runnin for a bus one night:::(.)I(h)(h)sstast
        couple of years ago(.)an me cracked (.3) un thats
        never been right but(.)hhh there's nothing at the
        back it's err┌:: itserr::like the cartilage
Dr:                  └(no::)
P:      I suppose(.)is it
Dr:     yeah
```

We enter the fragment as the doctor finishes examining the patient and returns to his desk to write a prescription. As he begins to write, the patient utters "see that one" and following a 1.4-second gap tells a story; the story concerns how the patient hurt her knee running for a bus. "See that one" serves as a preface to a story; it projects more to follow and gives a hint of what it might be—something relating to the other knee. As Sacks n.d. suggests, story prefaces give a flavour of the story and seek permission from the potential recipient to tell. In reply the potential recipient accepts or declines the opportunity to listen to and participate in the tale. In the case at hand it is interesting to note that the potential recipient, the doctor, produces no vocal response to the preface, yet a second or so later the patient spins her yarn.

As the doctor returns to his desk and begins to write the prescription, the patient remains standing. With "see that one" she points to the knee, thrusting her hand down and lifting her skirt to reveal the object in question. As she points, the doctor abandons writing the prescription and turns to the patient's face and follows her gaze to the knee.

Fragment 4:5   Transcript 2

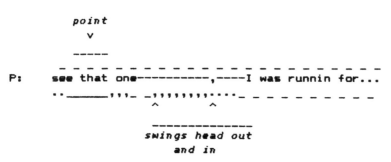

The doctor looks at the knee for a moment and then produces an exaggerated head movement. He turns away and returns his gaze to the knee, displaying a certain reconciliation to having to listen to the story. At the moment his gaze returns to the patient's knee she begins her story. Thus the initial realignment of gaze by the doctor passes unnoticed by the patient,[5] and the potential recipient, finding no story forthcoming, undertakes remedial action, recycling his shift in orientation in an exaggerated fashion. By turning towards the object the doctor reveals his willingness to receive the story and his preparedness to participate in the way encouraged by the speaker. And just as he uses the direction of the speaker's gaze to locate the object in question, so the speaker uses the recipient's orientation to discern whether he has focused on the knee.

Fragment 4:5 is different from the instances discussed earlier in that the recipient's gaze shift is more concerned with displaying cooperation with the projected future course of events than with attention to a course of action in which the speaker is at present engaged. Through his nonvocal actions both with and following the story preface, the doctor displays his preparedness to participate in and attend to the patient's story. It is the patient who encourages the recipient to participate in this fashion; through her preface and its accompanying nonvocal actions the patient invites the doctor to turn to her knee, and in so doing he displays his readiness to participate and cooperate with the telling of the story. The body movements of the doctor, with and immediately after the story preface, perform independent actions, particular forms of response to the preface and projected story. The patient not only elicits the doctor's cooperation but establishes a recipient who is looking at the knee and who can thereby use his examination to elucidate and assemble the sense of the story.

Rendering a gesture visible

In the preceding chapter I discussed the way in which a movement is used to attract another's gaze. It was noted that the action is designed to realign the other's gaze towards the face of the speaker rather than attract notice to movement itself. On some occasions, however, the speaker may wish to have another look not at his face nor at an object in the local milieu but rather at a gesture or a series of movements in which he is engaged.

Fragment 4:6   Transcript 1

```
Dr:    before you go: if you can:: (.3)remember
       (.4)
P:     When I went down in to Debenhams I an I felt so:
       aw::ful: (eh) I wen(.) I was coming up the steps
       li:ke this all the way up I felt (.3) terribly
       (.3)
P:     terrib⌈ly (.) really⌈you know
Dr:          ⌊yeh        ⌊yes
       (.2)
Dr:    No::::(.)its the knee itself(.)you've got some
       rheumatism there
```

After giving the patient some advice concerning how she should carry heavy objects, the doctor turns back to his desk to write a prescription. As he begins to write, the patient begins a story, a story concerning the difficulties she had walking up the steps at Debenhams. Accompanying the story is a series of movements through which the patient enacts these difficulties. She steps up and down on the spot as if hobbling up a staircase sideways. The movements illustrate her story and demonstrate how awful she felt. To comprehend the patient's difficulties and appreciate her suffering, the doctor needs both to hear the story and view the series of movements. The patient's movements appear to constitute what is referred to as "illustrative" or "iconic" gesture,[6] a gesture which visually represents a particular phenomenon and that frequently co-occurs with speech to perform a particular activity. In this example, without seeing the gesture, the recipient would be ignorant of the difficulties in walking up steps; without listening, a viewer would be ignorant of the setting of the difficulty and even what the movements are intended to represent. The speaker requires the recipient's participation as both a listener and a viewer of the events, yet as she begins her tale she is faced with a partner who is looking at the prescription pad, writing.

Fragment 4:6   Transcript 2

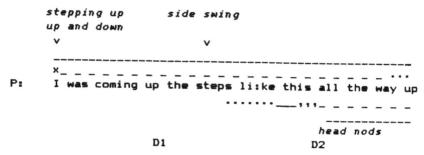

```
   stepping up        side swing
   up and down
      v                   v

   -----------------------------------------------------------
   x_ _ _ _ _ _ _ _ _ _ _ _ _ _ _ _ _ _ _ _ _ _ _ _ _ _ _ ...
P:  I was coming up the steps li:ke this all the way up
                       ........___,,,_ _ _ _ _ _ _ _
                               ----------------------
                                     head nods
               D1                    D2
```

The patient begins her illustration at the word "aw::ful:." There she turns sideways and begins to step up and down. The doctor continues to write. The self-correction "I wen(.)I was" following "aw::ful:" is perhaps a first attempt by the patient to encourage the doctor to look up.[7] If so, it fails and the patient continues her enactment unnoticed by the potential recipient. As the patient steps up and down for the second or third time she swings her bottom towards the doctor and his field of vision. As her bottom swings, the doctor abandons his activity and turns to look at the speaker's face. He finds the speaker neither looking at her recipient nor looking away but rather "looking at" her own legs and the movement in which they are engaged. Concurrently, as the doctor's gaze arrives at her face, the patient is uttering "this," a demonstrative referring to the movement. Before the word is fully uttered, the doctor turns from the speaker's face to her legs and there watches the movements which accompany her story.[8] The patient successfully encourages the doctor to view her difficulties in climbing the stairs at Debenhams.

Fragment 4:6   Drawings 1 and 2

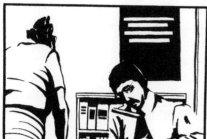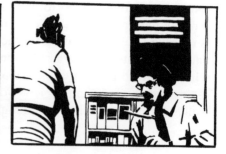

For many gestures which occur within talk, including illustrators and iconics, it is neither required nor encouraged that a co-participant should specifically view the movement itself. Much of the interactional work accomplished throughout movement is performed on the periphery of human vision, noticed but not seen, working alongside the business and involvement at hand. In fact, as we have seen elsewhere, for the accomplishment of many actions it is essential that the movement does not become the focus of visual or vocal attention. Yet on occasions a speaker, as in Fragment 4:6, may perform an activity in a way that requires the recipient not only to listen but also to watch a series of movements. In Fragment 4:6 it is almost as if the speaker, finding the potential recipient writing in the course of her telling the story, builds the activity in this fashion in order to harden up the obligations for his attention. Perhaps she even, on finding the doctor beginning to turn towards her, reshapes the utterance including "like this."

In the course of telling and enacting the story the speaker elicits the gaze of the potential recipient, first to the face and then to the illustration. The movement which elicits the gaze of the recipient is also part of the illustration. The bottom swing, though more exaggerated than earlier and later swings in the gesture, forms part of the overall movement, contributing to the appearance of climbing stairs with difficulty. The bottom swing, whilst being part of the gesture, serves to establish an audience, namely the doctor, for the illustration itself. Though part of the overall movement attracting the other's gaze is the servant of the activity in which it is embedded, it works both within and on behalf of the enactment.

In a recent paper Turner discusses what he refers to as "double duty utterances." These are utterances which perform more than one action.[9] He suggests:

> . . . there is no reason a priori to suppose that a single utterance is limited to the doing of a single action; it may well be that an utterance which provides an appropriate second pair part is simultaneously analyzable itself as a first pair part, in turn selecting a next activity for the co-participant to whom the floor is returned. (1976, p. 244)

In earlier chapters we have seen how a body movement may perform two distinct but interrelated tasks in the way Turner suggests. For example it has been found that the realignment of one person's gaze may be responsive to the gesture of a co-participant whilst encouraging the production or continuation of an utterance. The interactional responsibilities of the shift of gaze span out retroactively and proactively; it responds to the prior whilst eliciting a next action: a double-duty movement which operates sequentially back and forth. In a very different and more complex way the speaker's gesture in Fragment 4:6 also performs simultaneously two distinct but interrelated tasks. The movements serve to illustrate the difficulty of walking up the steps at Debenhams and form part of the activity of telling the story. The same movement, or at least a component of it, also elicits attention to the illustration itself. The movement establishes alternative sequential responsibilities for the co-participant. It encourages a reorientation by the doctor and forms part of an overall activity, on the completion of which the doctor is obliged to respond. More delicately still the same movement is working both to illustrate and work on behalf of the illustration, enacting the difficulties and simultaneously establishing an audience and thereby its own interactional significance.

Returning to some of the issues raised in the previous chapter concerning the design of movement, we can begin to discern how a gesture may be shaped to deal with concurrent operations of the same movement. In designing a movement to accomplish a certain interactional task, a person may at the same time produce the movement so as to accomplish distinct but related duties. Consequently the design of the movement has to take into account the considerations and contingencies which arise in the performance of both or all its actions. In Fragment 4:6 for example the speaker produces a movement which successfully encourages the doctor to realign his gaze. Like other movements which attract another's gaze it projects a part of the body towards the field of vision of the cointeractant and yet remains on the periphery. It stands out from the environment of goings-on both spatially and rhythmically; and in contrasting with the surrounding activity it draws the attention of the doctor to the speaker's face.

Simultaneously the movement forms part of an activity, which is illustrating the difficulty of climbing the stairs at Debenhams. The elicitation of the doctor's gaze is done as part of this overall activity and utilizes the resources provided through the illustration. The movement which elicits gaze is a bottom swing that also forms part of the stepping up and down. The patient does not break this activity but rather designs, whilst maintaining its shape, one of its components to stand out and contrast with the others. The bottom swing stands out spatially and rhythmically from the surrounding movements and serves to catch the doctor's eye, yet preserves the character of the illustration—providing the impression of walking up the steps with difficulty. The shaping of the gesture is accomplished in the course of its articulation; the patient, finding the doctor continuing to write the prescription, designs one of the components within the illustration to shift the way in which the recipient participates, thereby assisting the sequential significance of the activity itself. The illustration is the product of interaction between the speaker and the co-participant, its articulation and shape coordinated with consideration of the concurrent behaviour of the recipient.

A speaker may fail to encourage a potential recipient to participate in a particular fashion, such as to view a gesture.

Fragment 4:7 Transcript 1

```
Dr:    yes yes
P:     to get on that bus::(.)or in the car: (.2) its: a
       case of (uh) I can't breathe:: (.3) hum:::(.) you
       know (.)um::(.) an I'm all: trembly: an::┌(      )
Dr:                                             └are you
       allright when you get out of the bus or┌car
P:                                             └sweatin
Dr:    or is it?
       (1.2)
P:     it lasts until I get where I'm going
```

We enter this example as the patient is describing her complaint. She begins by setting the scene of the problem and then describes what happens: "I can't breathe::" and "I'm all: trembly:." Following an interjection by the doctor she tags on "sweatin." Coupled with the vocal description of the first two symptoms are a series of movements. Through these movements the patient enacts the difficulties she encounters when travelling in a bus or car. The patient adopts a facial expression of bewilderment and fluster whilst simultaneously trembling all over. As the patient sets the scene the potential recipient is reading the medical record cards.

Fragment 4:7 Transcript 2

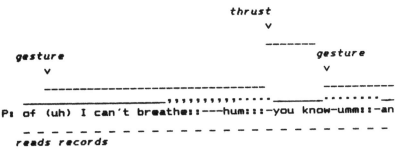

The patient begins her enactment with the vocal description of the first symptom. She thrusts her hands towards the doctor and then moves them both outwards in semicircles. As they swim outwards the hands begin to tremble, as do the patient's head and body. Starting to tremble, the patient turns away from the doctor and expresses her symptoms facially. As she enacts the difficulties she pauses and then utters "hum::::." Turning back to the doctor as her hands complete their semicircle, she finds him continuing to read the records, seemingly unaware of the elaborate performance conducted in his surgery. The patient utters "you know" and concurrently thrusts her head towards the doctor, a movement not unlike the action performed by the interviewer in Fragment 3:4. The package fails to elicit a response, and once again the patient enacts her symptoms. She thrusts her hands forward and then sweeps them around in semicircles; she trembles and once more assumes a facial expression of bewilderment and fluster. She returns her gaze to the doctor and completes the enactment towards the end of "um::," only to find that he is still reading the records. Sadly the performance once again passes unnoticed by the person for whom it is so elaborately conducted.

Fragment 4:7   Drawings 1 and 2

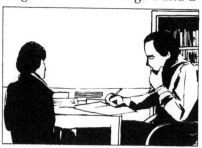 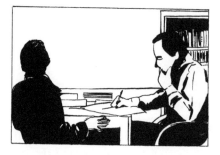

The speaker's enactments coupled with the articulation of the utterance are not only designed to illustrate the difficulties but simultaneously to encourage the potential recipient to attend to the performance. The patient pauses in the production of the utterance during both enactments, the pauses themselves perhaps attempts to encourage the somewhat recalcitrant recipient to attend. Between the two enactments the patient attempts to elicit a response with "you know" coupled with the head thrust. Moreover the enactments themselves both begin with the speaker thrusting both hands across the desk towards the doctor's field of vision, the area between his face and the medical record cards. And on top of all this, the trembling itself, perhaps the whole elaborateness of the enactments, may be concerned not only with simply illustrating the complaint but also encouraging the recipient to attend. It all fails.

On failing to encourage the doctor to participate visually, the patient describes the complaint vocally. As she returns her gaze to the doctor following the recycled enactment and finds her potential recipient still reading the records, the patient adds a further sentence to her utterance "an I'm all: trembly: an::( )." The patient describes vocally one, perhaps two, of the features displayed in her enactment, features which might otherwise have passed unnoticed. They may as well have for all the difference it makes, since in overlap with an additional symptom the doctor interjects a question. The question specifically addresses the scene and occasion of the trouble rather than the symptoms, shifting the focus of the discussion away from the particulars of the previous activity. And, as if in frustration, the patient tags on a further characteristic of the complaint at the first possible transition place[10] in the doctor's question, "sweatin" – a component which might also have been available in the enacted difficulties but one which again had passed unnoticed.

On failing to encourage the cointeractant to participate in the initial gesture, the speaker undertakes remedial action. She attempts to gather the other's attention and recycles the enactment. On its failure she adjusts the production format of the activity, describing rather than illustrating the symptoms. She adjusts the activity to the behaviour of the recipient and in particular designs it to cope with the form of participation and involvement the cointeractant may be prepared to provide.

Discussion: accomplishing the sense and impact of objects and activities

Pointing and showing are performed in a variety of ways, both vocal and visual. From within the small collection of examples discussed in this chapter we find persons encouraging others to notice objects in the local environment with gestures, postural shifts, rearrangements of dress, and a host of other means. In many cases these movements are packaged with aspects in the articulation of speech such as pauses that together encourage the recipient to look at something. Pointing and showing are sequentially implicative for an immediately following action; they encourage the recipient to turn towards and notice the object in question. They invite the cointeractant to reorientate his gaze and attention, an invitation that may be accepted or declined. Thus pointing and showing generate an interactional position where a co-participant is encouraged to produce a certain type of action; they work to invite a realignment of orientation to have an object noticed. And a person can inspect how the action is managed and, if the invitation is initially declined or unnoticed, take remedial action to encourage the recipient to accept.

An important aspect in pointing out an object and encouraging another to take notice of it is a person's line of regard. It will be recalled that in many of the examples discussed one person reveals an object to another and in so doing looks at the phenomenon. In many instances as the person points to the object he raises his eyebrows in exaggerated looking, as if looking at rather than simply away. The facial expression is not unlike surprise as described by Darwin:

> Attention, if sudden and close, graduates into surprise; and this into astonishment; and this into stupefied amazement. The latter frame of mind is closely akin to terror. Attention is shown by the eyebrows being slightly raised; and as this state increases into surprise, they are raised to a much greater extent, with the eyes and mouth widely open. The raising of the eyebrows is necessary in order that the eyes should be opened quickly and widely; and this movement produces transverse wrinkles across the forehead. The degree to which the eyes and mouth are opened corresponds with the degree of surprise felt; but these movements must be co-ordinated; for a widely opened mouth with eyebrows only slightly raised results in a meaningless grimace, as Dr. Duchenne has shown in one of his photographs. On the other hand, a person may often be seen to pretend surprise by merely raising his eyebrows. (1872/ 1934, p. 42)

A dramatic example may be found in Chapter 1 as Asia points out the camera to her father, but similar though less remarkable facial expressions occur in many of the examples presented in this chapter. The raised brows and staring eyes momentarily reveal that something has caught a person's gaze and warrants another's attention. The facial expression alone can be enough to encourage a recipient to search for an object, but more typically the raised brows and "open" eyes are used in conjunction with accompanying visual and vocal behaviour to display the noticeability of the object or event.

The exaggerated looking at serves to encourage another to realign the visual focus of his attention and also provides the information about where to look. Before bringing his gaze to bear on the object, the recipient may have little idea of what he is turning to and looking for. In determining where and what the object is, the cointeractant uses the direction of the other's gaze to organize the search. As he moves towards the object he may of course encounter a hand being moved towards him or leg being uncovered, but in the first instance he may only have the other's line of regard to follow. In many of the examples the cointeractant has frequently found and looked at the object in question even before it has been named or in any other way vocally referred to. A person's line of regard is used by another to discriminate the local environment and to determine an object which has been rendered noticeable and accountable.

Consequently we can begin to see the significance of an interactant gaining the gaze of another prior to pointing out an object. Both encouraging another to look elsewhere and indicating the location of the object are accomplished in part through a facial expression and orientation of gaze. As we noted in Fragments 4:3, 4:4, and 4:6, a prerequisite to realigning another's attention to an object may be eliciting his gaze to the face. In these instances it is found that a movement, coupled perhaps with a hesitation in speech, is used to elicit the co-participant's gaze to the face, and as it arrives the recipient is encouraged to turn elsewhere. Thus there is a string of four successive actions: the elicitation of gaze, followed by its reorientation to an object within the local milieu, where encouraging another to turn towards you serves as a prerequisite to shifting his attention elsewhere.

In the preceding chapters and now this, various fragments have been examined in which one person elicits the gaze of another. Even in instances where a person does not actually want the recipient gazing towards his face but at an object in the environment, he elicits the gaze to the face first if it is not already there. There is, of course, nothing intrinsic in the devices used to elicit another's gaze that determines that the other should turn towards the face. In fact one might imagine that some of the movements described in the preceding chapter and in this one might in themselves well attract another's notice to themselves; consider for example the leg tap or bottom swing. Yet in each case a between- or in-utterance pause, a gesture, a postural shift, or whatever brings the other into a face-to-face alignment with the speaker. Thus the examples in this and the preceding chapter suggest that there is a dominant form of response to perturbations or disruptions in the local, interactional environment: Turn in the first instance to the face of the other and then if necessary elsewhere. This convention holds whether the speaker is looking at the face of the potential recipient or not, and whether the speaker requires a face-to-face orientation or an object or movement to be noticed.[11] The organization of such responses, if correct, almost has the flavour of a basic human – even animal – reaction. The environment is monitored for sudden changes and disruptions and on their occurrence we turn and attend; interestingly, if it is another person producing the disruption in the first instance we turn towards his or her face.

In realigning another's gaze and encouraging him to take notice of an object or activity in the local environment, a speaker renders visible a phenomenon which might otherwise pass unnoticed. In each fragment the speaker not only encourages the recipient to participate in a certain fashion but brings to the other's attention a particular phenomenon. The specific appearance of the phenomenon, even its existence, may be unknown until it is actually looked at, the participant using the regard of the speaker to discriminate the environment and determine the object or activity in question. In generating the relevance of a phenomenon in the local milieu, the cointeractant is provided with a way of seeing, of perceiving the world at some moment in time. By turning his gaze upon the phenomenon the cointeractant reflexively constitutes the object or activity, assembling its occasioned sense in the very looking. In generating the relevance of a particular phenomenon, the speaker creates and topicalizes an object or activity, rendering it pertinent to the business at hand and momentarily bringing something to life through the shifting focus of attention.

As we have seen, realigning another's gaze through pointing and showing bears various relations to the talk with which it occurs. For example it has been observed that the very activity of encouraging another to look at an object or activity may itself be accomplished through pausing within an utterance and engaging in visual action. It has also been demonstrated that in various ways speakers may coordinate an utterance with a shift in alignment by a recipient. As we saw, an utterance may be withheld in its course and actually completed by the recipient looking at the object, or the speaker may delay speech until the recipient has turned to and looked at the object. And in Fragment 4:5 it was observed that before beginning a story the teller awaits the cointeractant's shift to the object which features in the tale. The speaker may articulate the utterance with respect to pointing and showing and withhold talk until he has successfully encouraged the recipient to realign his orientation.

The interrelation between the talk and the realignment of the recipient's gaze to an object or activity does not end there. In many of the fragments the recipient views the phenomenon whilst the speaker talks. In Fragment 4:6 for example the patient produces a series of movements that illustrate the problem mentioned in the talk. As suggested, the talk assists the series of movements, just as the movements are meaningful in relation to the accompanying talk. More precisely the speech and the movements are inseparable in the ways in which together they generate a particular activity; the activity achieves its sense and sequential significance through the vocal and visual. Realigning the recipient's gaze to view the legs is not simply concerned with eliciting a display of attention; rather it is a way of providing the recipient with the resources through which he can understand and thereby act on the activity of the speaker.

The same of course holds for many of the other examples. Consider the realignments of gaze in Fragments 4:3 and 4:4. In both cases the patients point out the complaint following the doctor's initiation of the business of the consultation. Realigning the gaze of the doctor to the complaint features in the activity of replying to the doctor's question. In fact in both cases the patient does not attempt to describe the physical appearance of the complaint, save perhaps for the "awfulness" of the spots; rather the description is rendered available through showing. Consequently the patient can proceed to add information which relies upon the doctor seeing the difficulty without needing to expand on the problem's appearance. In fact in both Fragments 4:3 and 4:4 the patient's vocal reply to the doctor's question does little more than refer to a problem, a problem which is already (at the beginning of the utterance) apparent to the doctor. Thus it is not simply that the speaker realigns the doctor's gaze and replies to him but that shifting the doctor's attention to the object is part and parcel of the reply. In pointing and showing the complaint to the doctor the patient provides his reason for the visit – the presentation of the complaint.

The interrelationship and interdependance of movement and speech in the articulation of the activities exemplifies the documentary method of interpretation described by Garfinkel (1967).[12] Drawing from Mannheim, Garfinkel demonstrates how the sense of action and activity is assembled through the mutual elaboration of an appearance and its presupposed underlying pattern, in a fashion not dissimilar to the functional significance of the constituent parts of the gestalt contexture discussed by Gurwitsch (1964). In the instances discussed earlier the recipient can use an inspection of the complaint to elaborate the sense of the accompanying talk, and the accompanying talk provides a way of interpreting and comprehending the actual appearances. Each is used to elaborate the other; the documentary method of interpretation informs both the articulation and the sense of the activity, movement and speech being reflexively embedded in each other and inseparable in the activity's accomplishment.

In this way one can begin to discern the significance of an interactant, say a speaker, attempting to establish a certain form of participation framework. This framework is not simply a means of interpreting the concerns of the speaker, a way for example of catching the gist of an utterance or the flavour of a story. It is more fundamental. The very production and understanding of the activity in which the speaker is engaged rely upon the potential recipient cooperating with the speaker and behaving in a certain fashion. At the beginning of the activity or actually in the course of its production, the speaker may encourage the recipient to orientate towards and participate in a particular way in the activity and thereby set the means through which it will be understood and produced. Failing to gain the recipient's cooperation may well lead to the activity passing unnoticed and/or the speaker refashioning how it is articulated. Recall Fragment 4:7 where the speaker illustrates her difficulties through gesture in the course of telling them. The speaker is unsuccessful in encouraging the doctor to attend to the illustration and reverts to an earlier production format, describing the symptoms vocally. Yet even that fails, and the patient finds that her activity passes unnoticed and gains little interactional significance. Production formats require participation frameworks to achieve the local and sequential implicativeness of actions and activities.

In the preceding chapter it was suggested that a speaker does not necessarily require the gaze of a recipient in producing an utterance and that many utterances are articulated with a recipient looking away. Speakers (or perhaps better participants) employ visual action to fashion responsibilities and obligations incumbent upon others within the perceptual range of the activity. As we have seen, movement prior to or during an activity can be used to elicit the gaze of one or more cointeractants, to encourage a display of heightened involvement, or as in the examples described here bring to the attention of others an object or movement in the local milieu. The ways in which interactants participate and sustain involvement are accomplished locally, step by step, utterance by utterance, the responsibilities and obligations of each person constantly being established and negotiated within the moment-by-moment articulation of body movement and talk, a partnership in the production of social actions and activities.

5. The physical examination

Licence my roving hands, and let them go, Before, behind,
between, above, below.

Donne 1633/1950, p. 88

Not merely do the practitioners, by virtue of gaining admission
to the charmed circle of colleagues, individually exercise the
license to do things others do not do, but collectively they
presume to tell society what is good and right for the individual
and for society at large in some aspect of life. Indeed, they set
the very terms in which people may think about this aspect of
life. The medical profession, for instance, is not content merely
to define the terms of medical practice. It also tries to define for
all of us the very nature of health and disease. When the
presumption of a group to a broad mandate of this kind is
explicitly or implicitly granted as legitimate, a profession has
come into being.

Hughes 1958, p. 79

Although defining a person as a technical object is necessary in
order for medical activities to proceed, it constitutes an indignity
in itself. This indignity can be cancelled or at least qualified by
simultaneously acknowledging the patient as a person.

Emerson 1970/1973, p. 362

In his essays on the nature of work and occupations Hughes develops
his classic statement concerning the licence and mandate of the medical
profession.[1] In everyday medical practice there is perhaps no clearer example of the legitimacy granted to the profession than the activities conducted by the doctor during the physical examination. In fact it is only
relatively recently that medical practitioners have been granted such a
broad licence to examine patients' bodies. In nineteenth-century England
the doctor would often place a small alabaster or marble figure on his
desk to enable patients to point to the area of the difficulty without having
to undergo physical examination.

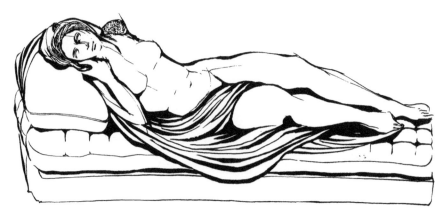

Nineteenth-century medical practitioners' figure.

In more recent years, however, the physical examination has become an integral feature of the medical consultation, so much so that patients are said to be disappointed if the body forgoes inspection. The practitioner's hands are granted licence reserved not even for the intimate, and patients are prepared to hand over their bodies for test and inspection. In so doing they are encouraged to relinquish some sensitivity over the body, to render it an object for analysis almost distinct from themselves. In the name of medical science and the management of illness they license the practitioner to perform activities few, if any others, may conduct and adopt a mandate as to how they should behave.

Whatever the licence and mandate granted to the medical profession, both doctor and patient have to accomplish the smooth running of the activity whenever it is necessary to conduct a physical examination. As Goffman (1959) and Emerson (1970) have pointed out, it takes no more than the slip of the hand to radically alter the definition of the situation, to disrupt the proceedings and transform the very nature of the event. Whatever routines the practitioner has developed for conducting particular types of examination have to be performed anew on each occasion, applied to the particular patient and his illness, and adapted to contingencies which may arise. For his own part, whether in distress or "merely" suffering the pangs of embarrassment, the patient in rendering himself as an object has to maintain a tight rein on his behaviour, cooperating with the activities of the doctor but not becoming too involved in the actions conducted upon him.

Consequently it is as if the participants, both doctor and patient, are subject to contradictory demands during the physical examination.[2] For the patient the concern is to attend and cooperate whilst remaining insensitive to much of the actual examination – the proddings, touchings, and the like it may entail – whereas the doctor has specifically to examine parts of the body whilst retaining some detachment, to treat the patient's body as an object yet maintain a concern for the patient as a person. It is within this complex array of demands and responsibilities that the work has to be accomplished, a situation requiring the utmost etiquette and diplomacy, and entailing a systematic and precise interactional organization.

Setting the scene

A doctor may be encouraged by the patient to conduct a physical examination. As in many of the examples discussed in Chapter 4, as patients describe their complaints they invite the doctor to inspect the relevant parts of their bodies. The doctor may respond by taking no more than a passing glance at the patient's complaint, but the invitation may lead to a fully fledged examination of the difficulty. In consequence of the point or showing, the participants realign their gaze and cooperate in rendering the visual manifestation of the complaint the central focus of attention. If talk continues during the examination, it is embedded in and organized around the activity of examining the complaint.

More frequently a physical examination is requested by the doctor.

Fragment 5:1   Transcript 1

```
Dr:    We 11 er::er::::::: shall I have a listen
P:        (          )
Dr:    to your ches:t heh heh                          undresses
P:                        yes::
       (7.5)
Dr:    thankyou
       (11.5)                                           dr
Dr:    just listen to the back please                  listens
       (8.5)                                            to chest
(_)    (ermm)                                           and
       (.)                                              back
Dr:    thhh(.)do you(r)::::(.)still feel a bit(.)
       tarry:
```

Presented in this way we can see the physical examination, listening to the patient's chest and back, as a chunk or episode of nonvocal activity bounded by talk, the interview of the patient. For the duration of the episode, talk is temporarily suspended, and is reintroduced the moment the doctor completes the activity. During the examination the participants remain visually orientated away from each other's face or gaze, the doctor conducting the activity and the patient being still and unresponsive to the various actions to which she is subject. For the doctor at least, the central focus of attention is listening and looking at the patient's chest and back, whilst the patient on the other hand is seemingly uninvolved. The obligations and responsibilities typically associated with face-to-face interaction are suspended and replaced by a framework of participation which provides for the smooth running of the physical activity, a framework in which the doctor and patient appear almost disengaged from each other's actions. As the doctor withdraws the stethoscope and the examination is brought to completion, the participants reorientate towards each other. They reintroduce talk and once more establish a state of mutual face-to-face involvement.

Unlike the examples discussed in Chapter 4, the physical examination in Fragment 5:1 is preceded by the doctor asking to listen to the patient's chest. The question (or better request) seeks the patient's permission to conduct the activity and her cooperation in its accomplishment. Permission is granted and cooperation given not simply by the "yes::" immediately following the doctor's request but through the patient's concurrent nonvocal activity. Even before the completion of the doctor's request the patient begins to remove the clothes from the upper part of her body and prepare herself for the proposed physical examination. Towards the end of the 7.5-second silence, the patient presents her chest, and the doctor, uttering "thankyou," begins to listen. Thus the physical examination, an episode of nonvocal activity conducted by one participant on the other, is preceded by an exchange through which permission is sought and granted and cooperation thereby achieved.

The structure is roughly analagous to the way in which stories are told, where one party needs to retain the floor for a series of interrelated utterances. As discussed in the previous chapter (Sacks n.d. is pertinent), the party who wishes to tell the story (conduct the activity) produces an utterance through which he seeks permission to tell the story and projects aspects of its character. In next position, the candidate recipient grants or declines permission for the story to be told. The exchange as in Fragment 5:1 prefaces the actual activity (if permission is granted); it projects the nature of the activity for which permission is sought and invites recipient cooperation. So, in contrast to pointings and showings where the examination may be coordinated with the speaker's invitation to look elsewhere, in cases such as Fragment 5:1 the examination is prefaced by an exchange in which the doctor seeks the patient's permission and formally initiates a shift in involvement.

A request to examine a patient may be declined, though in fact this rarely happens. In the corpus of data used for this research there are no examples of permission not being granted. General practitioners do mention that recent immigrants, especially Asian women, do refuse certain forms of physical examination. More often, however, though patients may indicate their willingness to undergo examination, they may actually withhold immediate cooperation or at times indicate that they are less than happy with the proposed course of action. Or for example a patient begins to undress but then successfully stalls, the doctor having to make repeated requests for the patient to present herself for examination. The patient's reply to a request to conduct a physical examination is also a basis for a show of embarrassment which briefly becomes the focus of discussion until the participants return to the business at hand: the patient preparing and presenting herself.

In granting permission for a physical examination the patient undertakes a course of action through which he makes himself available for inspection by the doctor.

Fragment 5:1   Transcript 2

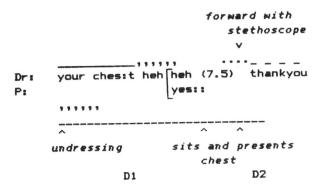

Drawings 1 and 2

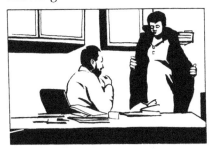
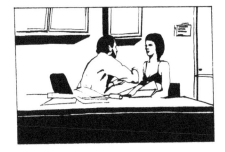

In this instance the patient prepares to undress during the doctor's request and by "yes::" she is standing and beginning to remove her clothes. As the patient stands, the doctor turns away from his co-participant and prepares his equipment, placing the stethoscope in his ears. Whilst the patient undresses both participants remain orientated away from each other, the doctor returning his gaze towards the patient only as she removes her final article of clothing. So too the patient, who whilst undressing never looks at the doctor, only turning towards him as she sits and presents her chest. Following the doctor's request to conduct the examination and during preparatory activity, the interactants temporarily disengage, shifting and displaying attention to distinct but related concerns, allowing each other to conduct activities which neither require nor demand the concern of the other. As the patient removes her pullover and presents her chest, the doctor turns towards her, stethoscope in hand, and the participants become once more orientated behaviourly towards a common activity.

The patient removes the clothes necessary to reveal the object in question and allow the projected activity to be accomplished. The patient presents her chest to the doctor, making it both visually available and physically within reach of the co-participant and the stethoscope. The patient reveals and aligns her chest so that it is at the correct angle, height, and distance for the proposed activity. The way the object is presented is designed with respect to the particular type of examination and the position and orientation of the doctor. The showing, the presentation of the object, allows the doctor to conduct the projected examination and encourages him to begin at a particular juncture.

In some instances the doctor may need to make additional requests so as to have the patient present the body in an appropriate way for the examination.

Fragment 5:2 Transcript 1

```
Dr:    Shall we just have a pee::p at your throat(.)today
       Rosemary
       (1.2)
Dr:    ○ can you o:pen wi::de
       (.2)
P:     hhhhh
Dr:    ooh my wor:d
       (.)
Dr:    ○ can you stick tongue ou::t
       (1.2)
Dr:    good
       (1.2)
Dr:    fi::ne
       (.8)
Dr:    in fa:ct(t) ac:tually(.)her tonsils an that look
       (.5) much more shrun:ken
```

At the end of the doctor's utterance through which he suggests peeping at the throat, Rosemary stands and presents herself in front of the doctor. As the doctor takes hold of a torch to light her throat she moves closer, making her throat available for inspection. As she holds herself facing the doctor she receives the specific instructions concerning the necessary bodily orientation for the examination, first to open her mouth and secondly, as he peers into her throat, to stick her tongue out. In responding to the doctor's requests Rosemary is able to present herself in such a fashion that she can become subject to the inspection of the doctor.

In both Fragments 5:1 and 5:2 the patient designs her bodily presentation not only in terms of the type of projected physical examination but also the orientation and visual activity of the doctor. The doctor's behaviour both during and following the request to examine the patient provides the resources through which the other can align the presentation of the complaint. In the following example the patient aligns herself with the doctor only to find him shifting position as he begins to conduct the examination.

Fragment 5:3 Transcript 1

```
Dr:    Can I jusht have a peep: ((whispered))
M:     hhh(.)hhh(hhh)
       (1.7)
Dr:    if we just look at you li::ke that
       (1.3)
Dr:    ohr:: ye:s::
       (2.2)
Dr:    hh(m) <I'm surprised < we haven't done anything
       about that ear::lier::
```

As the doctor asks to have a peep at the patient's ears, he raises both hands as if to receive his co-participant. As she stands, the patient moves her head towards the doctor so that it will fall midway between the two hands. The head and the hands move in unison towards each other, and just as the head is about to fall snugly into the open hands, the doctor changes position. He takes one hand and turns it towards the other, simultaneously shifting his gaze from the patient's face to the particular ear. As his hand alters position and moves towards the ear, the patient turns her head, presenting the particular ear to the doctor and his hand.

Fragment 5:3   Drawings 1 and 2

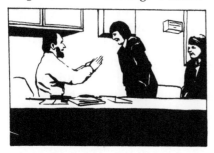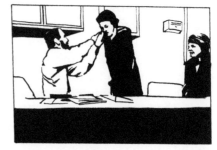

Yet as she presents her ear the doctor's hands once again alter their projected course and swing over the patient's head, both hands clasping the head and turning it face-on towards him. Even before the hands rest on the head, the patient begins to match the course of the hand and turns towards the doctor. And it is in this position that the examination is finally conducted, the doctor turning from ear to ear to determine the extent to which they protrude.

Fragment 5:3   Transcript 2

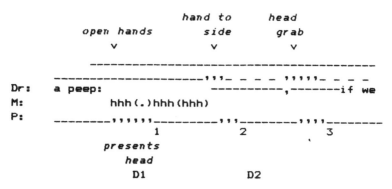

The patient makes a number of attempts to present the complaint to the doctor, each attempt being coordinated with the visual action of the co-participant. The patient uses the hands of the doctor and the alignment of his gaze to infer how she should place her body and in particular her head and ears. As the doctor's gaze shifts and his hands move she attempts to infer the presentation they demand and align her body accordingly. As they alter position for the third time the patient once again alters the way in which she presents herself for examination. In each case the patient uses the doctor's orientation and movements as a way of determining how the doctor wants her to participate during the course of the physical examination.

The doctor's request to conduct a physical examination, if granted, commits the patient to a course of action through which the appropriate body part is presented for examination. The nature of the complaint, the anticipated form of physical examination, and the doctor's nonvocal as well as vocal activity provide the patient with the resources through which an appropriate presentation is made. If preparatory activity such as undressing is required prior to the actual presentation, we find the participants temporarily disattending to each other's actions, only re-aligning their mutual involvement at the moment of presentation and inspection. Prefacing the physical examination with a request and granting of permission provides the participants with a stepwise progression into the realignment of involvement in the medical consultation. It provides for the collaborative achievement of a shift in the participation obligations incumbent upon the patient and doctor: movement out of talk into a mutually aligned episode of nonvocal activity.

Undergoing examination: attending to disattention

During the examination patients adopt a characteristic pose, a pose which is often maintained throughout its course. The pose is adopted by patients across a range of different types of examination, and it is relatively insensitive to the proddings, touchings, tests, and the like performed on the patient's body by the doctor. The following drawings provide a sense of the pose.[3]

Fragment 5:1 Drawing 3

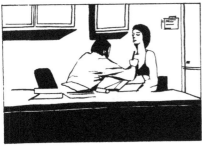

Fragment 5:4 Drawing 1

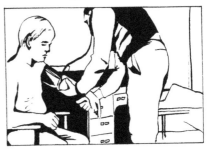

Fragment 5:5 Drawing 1

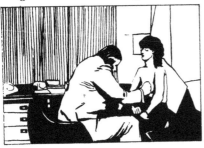

Fragment 5:6 Drawing 1

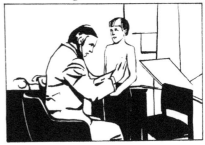

In each case it can be observed that the doctor is conducting an examination whilst the patient looks to one side, in many cases with the eyelids slightly lowered. Though the precise angle of the patient's orientation in relation to the examination and the doctor varies from case to case, it rarely moves further away than twenty-five degrees and typically remains just to one side of the co-participant. It is as if the patient is looking into the middle distance, away from the other, yet at no particular object in the local environment; the look casts its orientation to neither the foreground nor background but rather to an apparent middle domain. This middle-distance orientation is adopted at the beginning of the examination and then held. The patient rarely looks at the doctor, his face, or the area in which the examination is conducted. Whether the doctor is listening to the patient's chest, testing his blood pressure, tapping his body, or simply inspecting a difficulty, the patient looks to one side, seemingly inattentive to the proceedings. As the examination is brought to completion, the middle-distance look is abandoned, and the patient once again orientates towards the co-participant, taking note and attending to his action and activity.

Insensitivity

This middle-distance look, the pose adopted by patients during an examination, is insensitive to a range of actions performed by the doctor on the patient. For example whilst using the stethoscope the doctor may move the object around the patient's chest:

Fragment 5:1 Transcript 3 (listening)

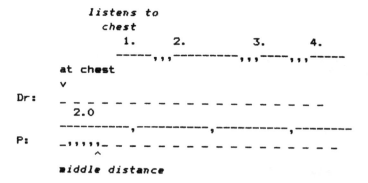

As the doctor approaches the stethoscope to the chest, the patient turns away, slightly raising her head and looking into the middle distance. Listening to the patient's chest involves moving the stethoscope from site to site over the patient's chest (and then her back). The doctor works his way across her chest and down towards the bosom. As he moves from site to site, the patient remains still and retains her pose. She provides no response to the doctor's actions, no receipt of or apparent attention to the activity in which he is engaged. Throughout the examination she remains seemingly unmoved and uninvolved, retaining her pose throughout its course.

In a blood-pressure examination the doctor wraps a rubber sock around the arm of the patient and then pumps it to apply pressure.

Fragment 5:4   Transcript 1

```
Dr:     Ill just:(.3)put this on::(.)an measure that first
        an then =
P:      =oh:ka┌y
Dr:           └then(.)then(.2)look at that all right
        <sorry its easier
        (1.2)
Dr:     to do it this way round
        (24.5)
Dr:     thats all right actually
```

Fragment 5:4   Transcript 2
(approx. 15.00 seconds into examination

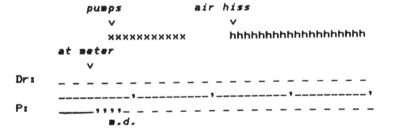

As the doctor wraps the arm, the patient turns away from the site of the examination and looks to one side with his eyes lowered. We enter in Transcript 2 as the doctor attaches the pumping mechanism and begins to inflate the rubber sock. The crosses mark the points where the doctor pumps, the row of *h*'s where he releases air from the sock. Throughout this part of the blood-pressure test the doctor is holding the patient's arm and looking at the meter attached to the sock. As the doctor attaches the pump the patient glances briefly at the arm. He then turns to one side and adopts a middle-distance orientation. This orientation is held as the doctor applies air to the rubber sock, neither the noise nor the pressure serving to alter the patient's pose. Similarly as the doctor ceases to pump and then releases the air from the sock the patient continues to look to one side with eyelids lowered. Both as the doctor prepares the arm for the test and whilst he conducts the operations the patient retains the middle-distance orientation, remaining unmoved and seemingly inattentive to the proceedings.

Patients assume and maintain the pose characteristic of examinations even under quite disturbing and potentially embarrassing circumstances. The following fragment is drawn from an examination in which the patient is undergoing an extensive investigation of her breasts and chest. The more detailed transcript is taken as the doctor begins to feel the side of the breast.

Fragment 5:5   Transcript 1

```
        (1.2)
Dr:     (eh.h) the pain was there:: wa⌈sn't it
P:                                     ⌊yes: err huh around
        there urm::
        (2.3)
Dr:     x x
        (.3)
Dr:     x x x (.2) x x x x x x x x x x x x x x x x x
        x x x x x x x x x x x x x x x x x
        (3.3)
Dr:     x x(.)x x(.)x x
        (.6)
Dr:     x x(.)x x(.)x
        (20.00)
Dr:     deep breath:
        (1.2)
P:      hhhhhh
```

Fragment 5:5   Transcript 2

```
        hand on breast
        v

        - - - - - - - - - - - - - - - - - - - - - - - - - - - -
              ._____'''_ _ _ _ _
Dr:     (1.2)(eh.h) the pain was there:: wa⌈sn't it
P:                                          ⌊yes: err huh around
        - - - - - - - - _-··_____-'''_ _ _
        ■.d.                                          ■.d.
```

As the doctor's hand lands on her breast the patient turns away and as in earlier cases raises her head slightly and looks into the middle distance. As he touches the breast the doctor questions the patient, and she briefly turns towards his face. As she replies she once again assumes the middle-distance look whilst the doctor feels around the area of pain. After a few seconds the doctor begins a different form of examination. He begins to tap his finger, hard enough to produce a knocking sound, on the patient's chest, beginning in the area of her shoulder and working across the chest and around one side of the breast. The crosses in the transcript represent the sound of the finger tapping the chest. As the doctor moves his hand from the area of pain to the shoulder, the patient turns and follows the hand. As it begins its new activity on the chest, the patient once again assumes the middle-distance look, gazing to one side of the doctor.

Fragment 5:5 Transcript 3

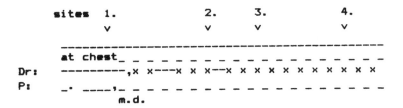

As in the earlier examples, as the doctor examines the patient by feeling around the area of pain or tapping different sites on her chest, the patient remains unmoved. Her gaze turned away, her body held firm, she produces no action in response to the doctor's feeling and tapping and provides no indication that she is receiving the doctor's actions or attention. During the brief exchange in which the doctor questions her concerning the location of the pain, she momentarily reorientates towards the speaker, returning to the middle-distance orientation before it is over. And even when the patient has to realign her body to enable a different form of examination to be conducted, she retains the middle-distance orientation, directing her gaze away from the doctor and the examination. In this way the patient subjects her body to another's scrutiny and becomes almost detached from the object under examination.

In the examples discussed so far, the patient is relatively inactive during the examination, rendering part of the body for inspection or test. During some physical examinations the patient is required to take a more active part, for example flex a leg to reveal distortion or, as in the following instance, take deep breaths whilst the doctor listens to the chest.

Fragment 5:6 Transcript 1

```
Dr:     othhh now I just want you < to take some deep
        breaths:: through your mouth alright?
        (1.2)
P:      hh ⌈hh
Dr:        ⌊right
P:      omm hhhhhhh
        (.5)
Dr:     again
        (1.2)
Dr:     out
P:      hhhhhhhhh
Dr:     and again
P:      ohh
        (1.0)
Dr:     out
P:      hhhhhhh
```

As the doctor asks the patient to take some breaths he moves the stethoscope towards the chest; it lands just following the completion of the utterance. The patient follows the stethoscope, and as it lands turns briefly towards the doctor. As he takes a deep breath the patient turns away from the doctor and gazes to one side. Save for one further brief glance towards the doctor, the patient retains this pose for the duration of the examination. As the patient responds to the doctor by taking deep breaths and the doctor listens at various points on his chest, the patient remains unmoved. He coordinates his breathing with the doctor's instructions yet remains visually orientated away from the doctor and the site of examination. The doctor encourages the patient to participate so as to reveal the object or function under examination, to follow the doctor's instructions but ignore the operations conducted upon the chest. The patient retains some involvement in the activity, enough to render the function hearable but not as a fully engaged participant in the business at hand.

Fragment 5:6 Transcript 2

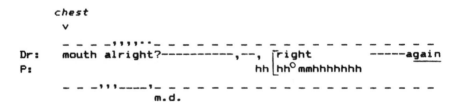

In each fragment therefore the patient turns away at the beginning of the examination and adopts the characteristic middle-distance look. From there on the patient remains unmoved throughout much of the activity conducted by the doctor as if there were passing unnoticed a business distinct from his own concerns. The operations performed upon the patient's body, whether applying pressure to an arm, taking soundings from a chest, or feeling a breast, fail to stir the patient into action. In looking more closely at the various examinations it can be seen that they consist of a series of interrelated actions performed by the doctor – successive tappings of the chest, listenings from site to site, or pumping of the arm. Each and every action conducted on the patient might in principle serve to elicit or encourage a response, some form of reaction to the operation on the body. No response is forthcoming. The patient withholds reactions to the successive actions performed on the body; each position where the patient might respond remains unfilled and unused. Any implication or interactional force the doctor's actions might suggest is ignored; the patient fails to act on the basis of the other's actions and temporarily becomes a minimal participant in the strip of activity.

It is not that patients are unaware of the operations to which they are subject during the examination; quite the contrary. They present their bodies and manage their behaviour in such a fashion that the doctor's actions seemingly pass unnoticed. They withhold response or, better, ignore the components of the examination which might elicit a reaction; they suppress any natural urge to react to the actions of the doctor. The patient disattends to the examination and achieves an apparent detachment from the proceedings by not responding. Though the patient is subject to the doctor's actions, he does not acknowledge or receive them. They neither elicit nor encourage subsequent action; they are treated as if devoid of sequential or interactional significance. By taking control of their bodies and behaviour in this fashion, patients render their bodies as objects; they temporarily transform themselves into phenomena under investigation. The middle-distance orientation and the unflinching body transform the very character of the patient as a person.

The physical examination is an episode of nonvocal activity which one party conducts on the other. The doctor secures or is offered permission to conduct the activity prior to its performance. Like telling a story, the physical examination is an activity familiar to one party rather than the other; it requires the cooperation of the recipient until its completion. In adopting the characteristic pose and remaining unmoved, patients provide an uninterrupted opportunity for the doctor to perform the activity. The type and timing of the actions performed on the patient by the doctor are coordinated with each other rather than synchronized with the actions of the patient. Even where the patient is encouraged to participate, it is to aid the appearance of the complaint and allow the examination to be conducted. The patient's actions do not fashion the form of the activity; they assist the examination but do not affect its structure. By participating as they do during the examination the patients render their bodies available but leave untouched the actual organization, an organization guided by medical practice and convention rather than by the momentary requirements of fully fledged interaction.

Sensitivity

If patients were simply required to make their bodies available and remain unresponsive during the examination, then one might expect to find behaviour other than the characteristic middle-distance pose. Patients could for example turn well away from the doctor or remain as they were but with their eyes closed. Yet neither happens, and in case after case we find the patient turning a little to one side, perhaps raising his head and lowering his eyelids. Though appearing inattentive, the patient does not abandon involvement in the activity altogether.

So for example, whilst adopting a middle-distance orientation and appearing inattentive to the proceedings, patients are able to cooperate with the doctor in bringing the activity to an end, often before any vocalization marks its completion. The withdrawal of the stethoscope or relaxation of a hand on the blood-pressure pump can have the patient reorientating to the doctor and once again fully engaged in interaction. It is also apparent that patients are sensitive to changes in the structure of the examination actually during its course:

Fragment 5:1 Transcript 4

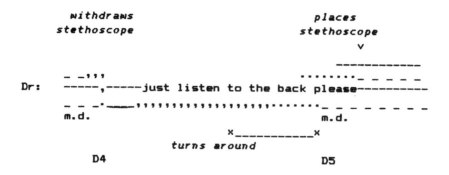

Here we find the patient, who has held a middle-distance orientation for more than eleven seconds whilst the doctor listens to her chest, turning first to the doctor and then briefly to the stethoscope. The change in orientation by the patient is responsive to the doctor beginning to turn away from the inspection site. As he then withdraws the stethoscope the patient turns from the doctor and watches his movements with the equipment. The positioning of the patient's shift of orientation first to the doctor and then to the equipment reveals her sensitivity to the behaviour of the doctor during the examination and her ability within the middle-distance orientation to monitor slight changes in the course of action. As the patient turns and watches the equipment, the doctor changes his orientation, beginning to move the stethoscope to one side; accordingly the patient alters her position, turning round before the request is complete and presenting her back to the doctor. Though facing in the opposite direction, the patient turns her head to one side and raises it slightly, lowering her eyes; she assumes once more what is akin to a middle-distance orientation.

Fragment 5:1   Drawings 4 and 5

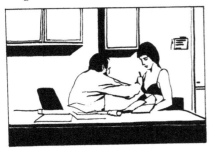 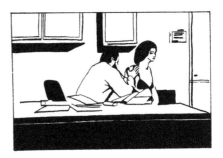

Consider another example, taken as the doctor prepares the blood-pressure test.

Fragment 5:4 Transcript 3

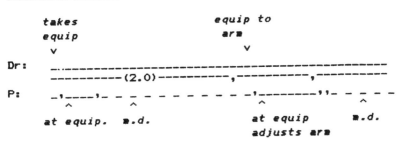

The patient assumes a middle-distance orientation as the doctor wraps the arm and prepares equipment; however, on a couple of occasions he turns and watches the doctor's hands. The changes in orientation are responsive to the doctor reaching out across his desk, breaking from the area in which he has been preparing equipment. In the first instance the patient resumes the middle-distance pose as the doctor's hand returns to its original position. In the second, the patient follows the hand as it goes to his arm and adjusts his position to allow the equipment to be fixed. As the doctor removes his hand from the arm the patient once more resumes the middle-distance pose.

A similar sensitivity is found during the actual examination. It will be recalled that in the following fragment the patient remains unmoved and retains a middle-distance orientation for much of the examination, even though subject to potentially disturbing actions.

Fragment 5:5 Transcript 4

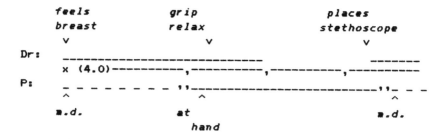

Here we find the patient maintaining her middle-distance orientation as the doctor taps the various sites on the chest and whilst he takes hold of and feels the breasts. At one point the doctor's hand begins to withdraw from the chest, and even before it has released the breast the patient turns and follows the hand. The slight relaxation of the hand appears to encourage her reorientation and renewed visual monitoring of the doctor. On withdrawing, the doctor takes hold of the stethoscope and then begins to listen to the chest. As he places it on her chest she adjusts her body to enable it to land flat on the area and simultaneously resumes a middle-distance orientation.

Fragment 5:5 Transcript 5

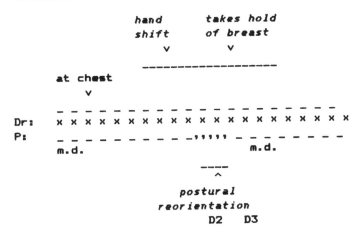

```
                hand        takes hold
                shift       of breast
                  v           v
                ------------------------
     at chest
         v
       _ _ _ _ _ _ _ _ _ _ _ _ _ _ _ _ _
Dr:    x x x x x x x x x x x x x x x x x x x x x
P:     _ _ _ _ _ _ _ _ _ _'''''  _ _ _ _ _ _ _ _
       m.d.                           m.d.
                         ----
                           ^
                     postural
                   reorientation
                      D2    D3
```

The second example is more delicate still. It is taken from a little earlier in the consultation as the doctor taps various sites on the chest. As the doctor's hands move progressively over the patient's chest, they near the patient's right breast. At one point one of the doctor's hands moves very slightly to one side, a moment or so later pushing the right breast to allow the tapping to continue in that area. The first, very slight, movement by the doctor's hand serves to attract the patient's gaze, and she momentarily abandons the middle-distance orientation. Seeing the direction of the doctor's hand movement, she begins to change her postural position, allowing the doctor easier access to her breast. The doctor's slight hand movement and the progressive course of the tapping allow the patient to anticipate the upcoming requirements and adjust her orientation even before the doctor's actions are complete. As his hand moves on to the breast she once more adopts a middle-distance orientation.

Fragment 5:5   Drawings 2 and 3

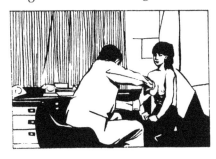
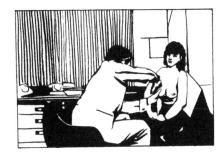

So far from being inattentive to the physical examination, the patient closely monitors the actions of the doctor and remains sensitive to changes in the articulation of the activity. The patient renders his body available for examination as an object of test and inspection, and whilst remaining unmoved and orientated away attends to the doctor's actions. The patient monitors the activity for any changes within its articulation which might require a shift in the fashion in which he is participating. For example the repositioning of a stethoscope may require a postural realignment, or the flex of a hand might suggest that the examination is drawing to a close and a face-to-face orientation is necessary. During the examination the patient monitors the environment of action, the successive operations of the doctor, so as to determine which actions should be ignored and which might implicate the way in which he should behave. The environment of action is discriminated with respect to the interactional responsibilities that the moment-by-moment articulation of the examination may suggest.

On the one hand therefore the physical examination requires the patient temporarily to transform himself into an object, to disattend to his own body and the actions performed upon him by the doctor. On the other hand the patient has to remain alive to the situation and closely monitor the actions of the doctor in order to determine and respond to the forms of participation they require. The middle-distance orientation is finely suited to solving these two almost contradictory demands. By not looking at the doctor the patient can appear interactionally, or, better, "communicatively," disengaged and show an inattention to the articulation of the activity. By turning away the patient can avoid placing the other under any obligation to respond or interact,[4] and by not watching the activity the patient can display trust and a lack of unreasonable concern in the details of the examination. Moreover by not watching the specific details of the activity the patient can perhaps diminish a desire to react to the doctor's moves, reactions which could well disrupt the accomplishment of the examination. In fact it has been observed in this data and elsewhere that children may often have to be explicitly encouraged to look away from the site of the examination, to avoid their potential reaction.[5] Turning away from the doctor and the area of the examination allows the patient to disengage from the doctor, to show a certain inattention to the activity, an involvement elsewhere; to transform himself temporarily into the object of test and inspection.

The middle-distance orientation allows the patient to maintain some visual attention to the performance of the activity whilst not watching the doctor or the examination (or be seen to be watching). In turning to one side and slightly lowering the lids, the patient can appear to be disattentive whilst continuing to monitor the actions of the doctor in a way that closing the eyes or turning right away would render impossible. In a way not unlike the design and recognition of movements used to elicit another's gaze (cf. Chapters 3 and 4), the patient adopts an orientation which enables him to monitor the actions of the doctor on the periphery of his vision, the corner of the eye. The middle-distance orientation allows the patient to monitor the accomplishment of the examination and render perceivable changes in the structure of the activity. The specific details of the doctor's actions may not be available to the patient in a middle-distance orientation; consequently shifts in the activity or sudden changes draw the patient's gaze so as to allow a determination of what is actually happening and the responsibilities which may be embedded therein. The middle-distance look relies upon an ability discussed in earlier chapters: the ability to monitor action and activity outside the direct line of regard and to be drawn by changes in the local environment of goings-on. During the examination this faculty, almost formalized in the middle-distance look, is put to the service of coping with competing interactional demands.

In passing, it is interesting that the middle-distance look does not occur only in the physical examination or the medical consultation. Anyone who has suffered the first few weeks of the services or even the school corps will recall how the middle-distance orientation plays an important part in parade and inspection. This aspect of military life is put to the service of melodrama in a film by Warner Brothers, *An Officer and a Gentleman* (1978), with the staff sergeant insisting on not being "eyeballed" and being looked at only on the periphery. In a rather different setting, visitors to auction houses may well have noticed how surreptitious bids will be accomplished from the floor by punters apparently uninvolved in the sale of a lot; and in the classroom teachers will recall the pupil who, appearing to keep an eye on the class, is receiving messages from a friend behind. The middle-distance look is a way of attending but not be seen to be attending, of being engaged but not engaged, of delicately monitoring the world on the periphery, the margins of visual involvement, ready for action should the occasion arise.

Finding the complaint and fixing the action

In the examples discussed so far the doctor and patient partially disengage for the duration of the physical examination. The request/grant format which prefaces the examination serves to suspend the relevancies and constraints of the turn-taking organization of talk, the doctor concentrating on the activity in question and the patient apparently disassociating from the business at hand and the co-participant. Yet during some physical examinations the doctor may need the patient to participate more actively in the examination; to respond and reply rather than assume a middle-distance orientation and become uninvolved. Such is the case where the doctor needs the patient's cooperation in order to find the area of the complaint. In the following fragment the patient moves in and out of "active" involvement during the course of the examination, and tension arises between the doctor's needs for assistance in locating the complaint and his co-participant's desire to disattend to the activity.

Fragment 5:7   Transcript 1

```
        (.5)
Dr:     This:: where it hurts::
        (.5)
P:      no:: (.2) over here:
        (.3)
Dr:     j:just a second(.)wait a minute
        (2.5)
Dr:     is:::very: pain:ful is it
        (15.00)
Dr:     Where is: it painful love (.2) top or at the back
        (.)hh
        (.6)
P:      here (.2) and: (.6) here
Dr:     an::here (.8) you can walk can't you
        (.5)
P:      I can't stand on it
```

This extract is drawn from a three-party consultation involving the patient (a teenage girl), her mother, and the doctor. The patient is a gymnast who has fallen from the bars and hurt her foot. The doctor places the girl's foot on his knee and in the course of the examination attempts to determine precisely where the area of difficulty is. We enter the scene as the doctor asks the patient where the foot hurts, and she replies, pointing to the position of the pain. Following the exchange the patient attempts to withdraw her foot, but the doctor clasps it back to his knee and continues to search for the precise location of the pain. After nodding a reply to whether it is painful, the patient adopts the characteristic middle-distance pose.

Fragment 5:7   Transcript 2 (6.0 seconds into examination)

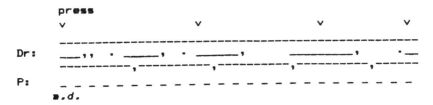

With the foot on his knee, the doctor presses lightly over its surface, intermittently glancing at the patient's face. Unlike the tappings and touchings found in earlier examples, in Fragment 5:7 the doctor's examination is an attempt to elicit a response from the patient, a response which would indicate whether or not his fingers have identified the precise area of difficulty. As he presses on the foot he turns to the patient's face seeking to detect a reaction, the intermittent glances themselves encouraging the patient to respond, to display recipiency, and to signal where the difficulty is. Yet neither the surface pressings of the foot nor the intermittent glances encourage the patient to participate as an active interactant; she steadfastly maintains her middle-distance orientation, and, following successive attempts to elicit a response, the doctor once again asks her where the difficulty is.

Fragment 5:7   Transcript 3

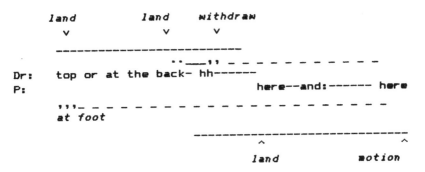

Both utterances are accompanied by and rely for their sense on movement. As the doctor asks where it is painful he places his thumb and forefinger on two sites of the foot; the determination of the "top" and the "back" being rendered through the position of the thumb and forefinger. As she replies the patient places her hand on her foot. It lands and she utters "here" and then moves her hand to a different site on the heel. The hand lands on the foot for a second time and the patient begins a circular motion uttering "here." The hand then quits the foot and returns to base. In the course of the gesture the patient produces vocalizations "here (.2) and: (.6) here" that are staggered. They are positioned in terms of the movement they accompany and break the movement into two distinct parts: the initial foot touch and the following circular motion. The vocalizations accompany and mark certain moments in the articulation of the gesture. They locate within the movement precisely where the pain is, serving to produce actions within the overall activity of the gesture.

Fragment 5:7   Drawings 1 and 2

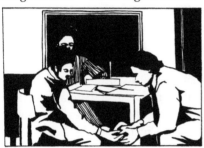 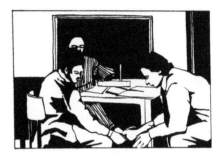

The package of utterance and movement is even more subtle. The two points displayed in the gesture involve different forms of action. In the first the patient holds the foot with the thumb and forefinger; in the second the patient strokes the upper part of the heel with her fingers in a semicircular motion. "Here (.2) and: (.6) here" within the movement not only mark and produce two distinct points but differentiate these points, revealing one as a specific location and the other as an area. The points of the complaint are displayed in and through the movement and vocalization as both regionally and qualitatively different.

Elsewhere I have remarked upon the way in which movement and speech may be packaged together to perform a particular action and activity. As Fragment 5:7 reveals, the package may not simply entail the co-occurrence of a certain vocalization and movement but rather a complex interweaving of the vocal and visual so as to determine the particular kind of action or activity. In this example we can begin to discern how speech may accompany movement and be coordinated with a gesture so as to fix the moments of its actions. The actual vocalizations are positioned with consideration to the articulation of the movement, fixing just the elements of the gesture which are showing the position of the complaint. Consequently, even though the patient's movements as a whole – the hand's journey to and from the site and the touchings – are visually available to the recipient,[6] it is the points fixed by the hand and accompanying vocalization which achieve performative force. Within the overall activity the speaker produces just the moments and movements which are of interactional significance, which address the injury and implicate the complaint's examination.

In Fragment 5:7 the patient is encouraged to retain involvement in the physical orientation and actively assist the doctor in locating the area of difficulty. The doctor in the course of the examination makes successive attempts to have the patient participate by locating the complaint. The patient drifts into a middle-distance orientation whilst the doctor struggles on, trying to determine the specific location of the complaint. Finally the doctor drags the patient back into a state of mutual engagement by asking a question which requires the patient to articulate an action both vocally and visually. Unlike earlier examples where part of the body is presented and treated as if it were an object, in Fragment 5:7 the patient is encouraged to retain attention and sensitivity to the body part in question. The patient is required to receive and respond to the actions performed on the body by the doctor, to subject herself to inspection and maintain involvement in the activity at hand.

Discussion and a note on embarrassment

The physical examination entails a strip of technical activity performed on the patient by the doctor. The technical details of the activity, the medical conventions and procedures which underlie the physical examination, may be unknown and unavailable to the patient, as may the ways in which the doctor sees and comprehends the complaint during its professional inspection. In designing and conducting the examination the doctor relies on information provided by the patient – the location of the trouble, the suffering it causes, its progression over time, the patient's perspective and knowledge – to inspect and interpret the complaint in specialized ways and apply the science.[7] In the context of the details of a particular complaint and its examination, the doctor performs a technical activity which has a structure and organization determined by some set of medically warranted conventions and procedures.

Whatever the technicalities of the activity, the doctor requires the co-operation of the patient in order to conduct the physical examination. At its most basic the doctor needs to gain the floor for an uninterrupted strip of activity and retain the patient's cooperation until the proper completion of the examination. The patient is required not only to engage in the relevant preparatory activity, such as undressing and presenting the complaint for inspection, but also in participating in an appropriate fashion throughout the examination, a fashion which allows and assists the doctor to follow the technical conventions. Not surprisingly therefore, the physical examination is prefaced by a sequence through which the doctor gains permission to conduct the activity and secures the cooperation of the patient in its performance. In agreeing, the patient commits himself to present the complaint for examination and assumes the responsibilities involved in being an object of inspection. In this way the doctor secures the opportunity of conducting an activity the organization of which is determined by medically warranted conventions and procedures rather than by the patient's in-course responses.

The practitioner's licence to conduct the physical examination rests in part on the management the doctor is able to provide to the patient. Following the physical examination and perhaps further inquiries, the doctor is expected and obliged to form some kind of assessment and if necessary offer treatment for the patient's complaint. Unlike the completion of, say, a story, which is a focus for recipient appreciation, second stories, and the like (cf. Sacks n.d.), completion of the physical examination calls for some comment or assessment by the practitioner. In case after case as the examination is brought to an end the doctor produces some form of assessment, not infrequently a diagnosis, and goes on to discuss how the complaint should be managed. In cases where assessments are not immediately forthcoming on the completion of the examination or are temporarily suspended through further inquiries, we find the patient pressing the doctor for a comment and even diagnosis.[8]

Earlier chapters addressed the ways in which an interactant may attempt to gain another's attention or his participation in an activity. In so doing the interactant, typically the speaker, does not only establish the other's participation in the activity but encourages the recipient to treat the activity sequentially in a fashion the recipient may not have chosen. With the physical examination we are faced with a very different situation. An interactant is encouraged, in large part, not to display attention to the proceedings, to ignore much of what goes on, and to avoid showing receipt of the particular actions. Rather than actively seeking heightened participation from the cointeractant, the doctor attempts to minimize the performative impact of a range of actions and not have them treated sequentially or responded to by the patient. The patient's in-course responses could undermine the internal organization of the activity and disrupt just those technical details which render the physical examination the activity that it is.

In her excellent study of the gynaecological examination (1970) Emerson discusses how participants attempt to sustain a mutually achieved definition of the situation in the face of potentially contradictory demands and interpretations. One particular area examined in her study is the ways in which doctor and patient cope with rendering the body as an object whilst retaining the integrity and humanity of the person. The middle-distance orientation, the insensitivity yet attention to the business at hand, involved whilst not involved, similarly reflect and attempt to solve the contrast between behaving as a person yet temporarily being treated as an object. Whilst rendering himself as an object, the patient remains a participant; whilst presenting the body, the patient retains control of the body; whilst not receiving, the patient is attentive to changes in the participation requirements. The contradictory demands of being a person and an object, of being involved yet uninvolved, are an essential part of the physical examination and fundamental to its smooth running and practical accomplishment.

Thus in discouraging patients to attend to and receive actions within the physical examination, it is not that doctors desire the patient temporarily to suspend altogether his involvement or participation in the business at hand. The doctor requires the patient's continued involvement to render his body available and present it in an appropriate manner and to make the required adjustments in its presentation during the course of the examination. Consequently, whilst disattending to the activity performed on their bodies, patients are required to strictly monitor the course of action and discriminate what and what may not be relevant to their presentation and participation. The middle-distance orientation provides a solution to the almost incompatible demands on the patient during the physical examination. It allows the patient to appear and remain seemingly uninvolved in the activity whilst providing the opportunity to monitor the doctor's actions for any shifts in participation they might suggest or require.

The middle-distance look and the fashion in which patients present their bodies for inspection are pertinent to the issue of embarrassment.[9] In principle one would consider that the physical examination is fraught with potential embarrassment, embarrassment which if manifest could disrupt the very accomplishment of the activity. Dressing and undressing, the revelation of intimate parts of the body, the feel of another's hands and the attention of his look might all give rise to embarrassment, perhaps even disturb and distress. Yet a search through many hours of video recordings of the physical examination reveals little evidence of embarrassment and consequent problems. Rather than assume that neither patient nor doctor suffers embarrassment or that the physical examination does not hold such potential for disruption, it would seem more reasonable to suppose that patients manage potentially embarrassing moments and keep them from becoming manifest and disrupting the activity. We find for example that doctors do not watch patients dress or undress, shifting their attention to an activity at hand or sustaining a face-to-face orientation whilst continuing to talk. Moreover doctors do not simply look at the patient's body whilst it is disrobed, but rather conduct an activity a feature of which is visibly inspecting part of the body. Frequently the lookings are accompanied by technical uses of the hands in the area of visual attention; the looking is warranted as part of the activity in the name of determining the nature of the illness.

Embarrassment, however, does not simply derive from the potential, actual or not of having another inspect a part of your body or see an activity in which you are engaged. Rather it derives from your seeing another seeing those objects and activities. It is the mutual recognition that may give rise to embarrassment: seeing another see you in a certain fashion. Consequently it is found that the patient avoids viewing the other during moments of potential embarrassment; even male patients removing only a shirt turn away from the doctor whilst undressing. And during the examination itself the middle-distance orientation again provides a solution, here to the difficulties that may arise as a consequence of another seeing and inspecting one's body. It allows the patient to avoid watching the doctor during the examination whilst keeping an eye on the proceedings. More important, it provides a way of not having the other see you seeing him look at your body; of apparently disattending his attention. By avoiding the gaze of the other and that mutual recognition it is possible to manage the potential embarrassment that lingers in a physical examination.

However, embarrassment is not necessarily a phenomenon that persons wish to conceal. In fact if a person does not show embarrassment in certain circumstances, the consequences for the assessment of his or her moral integrity may be grave. Decorum can require a person to be embarrassed and thereby display sensitivity to the contingencies at hand and to the moral order. Though sadly there is not the space here to demonstrate the point, it is worth noting that where embarrassment does emerge in the consultation and in particular in the physical examination, it appears that both patient and doctor actively collaborate in its manifestation. Far from attempting to suppress the expression of embarrassment, they mutually encourage its demonstration, producing temporarily a distinct episode, a shift in involvement in which embarrassment bubbles over and subsides, doctor and patient quickly returning to the main concern at hand and instantly banishing any further expression of their mutual sensitivities.

As Hughes points out, members of the public not only grant the medical profession a licence to conduct activities that others may not perform but provide a mandate by behaving in such a fashion that the activities may be performed as smoothly as possible. On every occasion, the profession is either invited to conduct particular activities or seeks the permission of the patient, and in granting permission the patient agrees to collaborate in assisting the performance of activities reserved for the very few. In the physical examination patients present their bodies for inspection and in so doing relinquish a little of their selves, their right to be treated as fully ratified participants in the interaction. Yet even here in the rendering of a body for inspection, the professional has to rely upon the ordinary abilities of the patient to disassociate yet maintain attention to the business at hand. However technical the examination, it has to be articulated in such a way that the patient can comprehend its local organization and thereby cooperate in its performance.

6. Taking leave of the doctor

In face-to-face interaction, a whole range of physical doings and positionings, ruled out by the proprieties of maintaining a show of attention and interest, become available and/or required upon termination, for example, those related to leave-taking. In so far as the actions that may be occasioned by termination of the conversation require preparation, there is use for a place in the conversation to prepare for actions that should follow its termination in close order.

Schegloff and Sacks 1973/1974, p. 261

On when to go – your exit cues are many. They range from clear-cut closing remarks, usually in the form of a "thank you for coming in," to a vacant and preoccupied stare. But in any case they should come from the interviewer. It should not be necessary for him to stand, abruptly; you should have been able to feel the goodbye in the air far enough in advance to gather up your gear, slide forward to the edge of your chair and launch into a thank-you speech of your own. Nor should it be necessary to ask that embarrassing question, "Am I taking too much of your time?"; if that thought crosses your mind, it's time to go.

Esquire Etiquette 1953, p. 59

As we have seen, the medical consultation, like any other form of social interaction, relies upon the participants maintaining some semblance of mutual involvement and thereby coordinating their actions and activities. The interactants encourage each other to attend and participate in certain ways. They accomplish various tasks and implicate subsequent action and activity. Bringing the consultation to an end entails finishing with the topic of the encounter and disentangling the participants from a web of interactional commitment.[1] In ending the consultation doctor and patient have to step from a state of mutual involvement and orientation and accomplish an inattention to each other's actions; they have to realign their responsibilities and obligations and rid their actions and activities of interactional consequence.

Ending the consultation entails bringing the business to a satisfactory conclusion: providing the patient with appropriate management for a particular complaint. On discovering the problem from which a patient is suffering or how a certain problem has developed, the doctor is obliged to offer some form of help to the patient with whom he is faced.[2] The last few minutes of the consultation frequently involve the doctor writing prescriptions, telling the patient what he intends to do, and arranging future appointments. The patient receives advice, sick notes, prescriptions, and the like, and talk is brought to completion. The end also involves, as do many face-to-face encounters, the participants breaking each other's presence so that they are no longer interactionally or physically available. The process of taking leave is thoroughly bound up with the doctor's and the patient's movement out of the business of the consultation and a state of mutually coordinated talk.

In the general-practice consultation, as with other forms of professional–client interaction, it is generally the patient who quits the doctor. The doctor remains seated whilst the patient stands and leaves the surgery. Taking leave of the doctor involves the patient in a course of action, an activity through which co-presence is broken with the cointeractant. From the start, the activity projects a trajectory of action, a series of moves through which the face-to-face orientation is dismantled, and mutually coordinated interaction is brought to an end. The series of movements through which patients break co-presence are repeated from consultation to consultation; they form a standard episode of nonvocal action, a recurrent activity. The following couple of drawings capture just two slices of the activity.

Fragment 6:1   Drawings 3 and 4

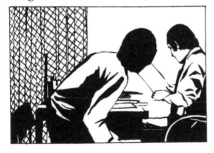 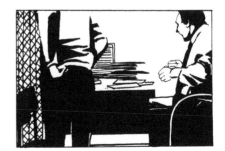

It might be thought that patients begin this episode of nonvocal activity after they have finished talking with the doctor, or even that quitting the surgery is a relatively haphazard activity begun whenever one is ready to go. Neither appears to be the case. By the time talk has finished, the patient is well on his way, often walking out of the surgery door. Taking leave of the doctor is begun during the consultation itself whilst the doctor and the patient are still speaking. And, far from this pattern being idiosyncratic, the patient begins to take leave of the doctor time and time again at a particular position in the course of the interaction.

Fragment 6:1   Transcript 1

```
Dr:     Now have you got enough medicine and so on?
        (.2)
P:      err it's finished ⌈with
Dr:                       ⌊it's finished you(.)ah you'd like
        some more (.4) medicine?
        (3.4)
Dr:     and the tablets:::?
        (.2)
P:      err also finished
Dr:     uh huh
        (26.00) ((writes prescription))
Dr:     O.kay Mister Hough I'll send that (.8) off: (.3) or
        you take it down (1.2) to the reception
        (.3)
Dr:     and the girls will send it off
        (.3)
P:      Thankyou very much
Dr:     O.kay
P:      Thankyou again
```

This fragment captures closing moments of a lengthy consultation in which the doctor and patient discuss the possibility of the patient suffering a duodenal ulcer. The doctor inquires whether the patient needs any more medicine and tablets, and he then writes a prescription. Turning to the end of the fragment, it can be found that the consultation is brought to completion through the exchange of two utterances, one by the doctor, the other by the patient:

Fragment 6:1   Transcript 1a

```
Dr:     O.kay
P:      Thankyou again
```

Through this exchange of utterances the doctor and patient provide an orderly basis for the termination of talk and the end of the consultation. As Schegloff and Sacks (1973/74) suggest, this form of utterance sequence, the "terminal exchange," allows the interactants systematically to lift the relevance of the turn-taking organization of talk so that "one speaker's completion will not occasion another speaker's talk, and that will not be heard as some speaker's silence" (p. 237). The exchange of utterances which lifts the relevance of turn taking and brings the consultation to an end does not occur anywhere in the developing course of the consultation, but is systematically placed in a properly initiated closing section (cf. Schegloff and Sacks 1973).[3]

Fragment 6:1   Transcript Ib

```
Dr:    O.kay Mr. Hough I'll send that (.8) off: (.3) or
       you take it down (1.2) to the reception
       (.3)
       and the girls will send it off
       (.3)
P:     Thankyou very much
```

In the data at hand it is the doctor's turn at talk beginning "O.kay Mister Hough" and the patient's reply that pave the way for the exchange of utterances that brings the consultation to a close. The doctor's utterance is positioned just as he finishes writing the patient's prescription. It proposes a course of action for the patient relevant to his complaint and its management. Within the utterance the doctor passes the patient a couple of pieces of paper, one the prescription, the other an appointment card for an X ray. The doctor's utterance coupled with the exchange of objects serves to provide the patient with the management of the complaint; they provide a service, given the patient's reason for the visit. In treating the patient for the complaint, the doctor proposes the end of the business of the consultation, at least for now.

The utterance provides the patient with the opportunity in next turn not only to agree to the recommended course of action but to accept or decline the proposed end to the business at hand. In this instance the patient accepts, with "Thankyou very much," and the acceptance allows the doctor to initiate a sequence of utterances which leads to the completion of talk and the end of the consultation. Thus the doctor's utterance beginning "O.kay Mister Hough" coupled with the passing of objects initiates a course of events which moves the consultation out of the business or topic at hand through to its close. The consultation is brought to an end through a four-utterance section which establishes the completion of the business of the interview and progressively brings the state of talk to a mutually agreed end. The consultation's end is achieved by and through this closing section.

Breaking co-presence and the end of the consultation

Taking leave of the doctor typically begins before the terminal exchange but in the closing section of the consultation.

Fragment 6:1   Transcript 2

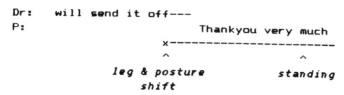

```
Dr:    will send it off---
P:                              Thankyou very much
                    x-----------------------------
                    ^                        ^
              leg & posture            standing
                 shift
```

At the completion of the doctor's utterance, actually before he begins to reply, the patient begins to take his leave. He swings his right leg out and posture-shifts forward: He adjusts his hands and thrusts himself upwards. By the end of his reply the patient is standing and turning to quit the surgery. In Fragment 6:1 the course of action through which the patient breaks co-presence begins at the completion of the utterance in which the doctor proposes the end of the business at hand, topic completion. As the patient takes his leave, he responds to the doctor, accepting the proposal to end the consultation.

Fragment 6:2 Transcript 1

```
          (16.00)
P:        It's only once that's all
          (2.7)
Dr:       O.kay
P:        Thanks alot
          (.5)
Dr:       Thank [you
P:              [Thankyou very much
Dr:       Bye bye
          (2.0)
P:        (Right)
          (.3)
P:        Bye
```

During the (2.7) sound gap the doctor is writing a prescription, and as he utters "Okay" he rips it from the pad and passes it to the patient.

Passing the prescription and uttering "Okay" serves to propose the completion of the business of the consultation, and provides the patient with the opportunity in next turn to accept or decline. The patient accepts with "Thanks alot" and simultaneously begins to take the doctor's leave.

Fragment 6:2 Drawings 1 and 2

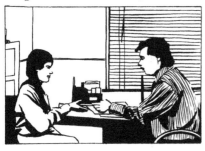 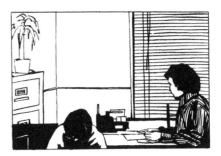

```
        D1              D2
Dr:     O.kay
                Thanks alot------
```

The following fragment is drawn from the end of a multiparty consultation involving a mother, her two children and a baby, and of course the doctor. After dealing with the children's complaints, colds and coughs, the mother and doctor discuss the underlying cause, their appalling housing conditions.

Fragment 6:3 Transcript 1

```
M:      The tiles are off the roof(.)there's a leak in his
        bedroom ᕁhhh got a big hole in our bedroom (.2)
        ceiling
Dr:     yeah
        (.8)
Dr:     I'll write (.2) I'll write them a letter
M:      Oh than⌈ks
Dr:        ⌊O.kay then
M:      Thanks very much doctor
Dr:     O.kay
M:      Thank you
M:      Bye bye
Dr:     Cheerio
P1:     By bye
Dr:     Chee⌈rio
P2:        ⌊bye
        (.5)
M:      Bye thankyou
P1:     Thankyou
```

The mother's description is acknowledged by the doctor with "yeah," and talk between the participants momentarily lapses. The silence is broken by the doctor, who repeats an offer he made earlier – to write a letter to the council. The utterance is treated as proposing the end of the business of the consultation, and the mother accepts in next turn with "Oh thanks." As she utters "Oh thanks" the mother begins to leave, rocking forward to stand. As she begins to stand, the two children, who are standing close to the doctor's desk, turn away and also begin the process of leaving.

Fragment 6:3 Transcript 2

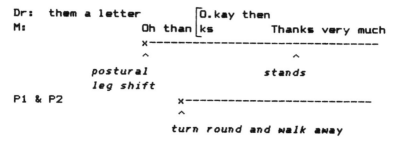

```
Dr:    them a letter           ⌈O.kay then
M:                     Oh than⌊ks          Thanks very much
                      x------------------------------------
                      ^                    ^
            postural                 stands
            leg shift
P1 & P2                           x----------------------------
                                  ^
                    turn round and walk away
```

In Fragment 6:3 therefore, as with earlier examples, breaking co-presence is coordinated with the turn-by-turn organization of talk and the progressive movement out of the business of the consultation. In each case the patient(s and parent) begins to quit the presence of the doctor precisely at the completion of a particular turn at talk. As he accepts the doctor's proposal to end the business of the consultation, he takes leave of the doctor and prepares to quit the surgery. Breaking co-presence has an almost turn-like character, fitted within the utterance-by-utterance structure of the talk and coordinated with consideration to the prior utterance and the mutually agreed end of the topic at hand.

The behaviour of the participants prior to one successfully taking the other's leave may also reveal an orientation to utterance and topic completion. For example consider Fragment 6:1 and the doctor's proposal to end the business at hand: "O.kay Mister Hough . . ." The utterance consists of a number of "turn constructional units," each of which marks a point at which speaker transition might properly occur. As Sacks, Schegloff, and Jefferson suggest:

> There are various unit-types with which a speaker may set out to construct a turn. Unit-types for English include sentential, clausal, phrasal and lexical constructions. Instances of the unit-types so usable allow a projection of the unit-type underway and what,

roughly, it will take for an instance of that unit-type to be completed. Unit-types that lack the feature of projectability may not be usable in the same way. . . . For the unit-types a speaker employs in starting the construction of a turns talk, the speaker is initially entitled in having a "turn," to one such unit. The first possible completion of a first such unit constitutes an initial transition-relevance place. Transfer of speakership is coordinated by reference to such transition-relevance places, which any unit-type instance will reach. (1974/1978, p. 12)

In Fragment 6:1 "O.kay Mister Hough" and "I'll send that (.8) off:" are turn constructional units and in principle suggest transition-relevance places, places at which Mr. Hough could have spoken. However, the doctor produces these and the following unit "or you take it down" so as to project more to follow. The units are produced without the falling intonation characteristic of turn or topic completion; moreover throughout these units and across their transition-relevance places the doctor is engaged in various nonvocal activities, gesturing and passing notes to the patient. In contrast, the turn constructional unit ending "reception" can be heard and seen as a place where the doctor is bringing the utterance to completion. It has a falling intonation, and the doctor moves posturally away from the patient with "reception."[4]

Fragment 6:1 Transcript 3

```
        Posture shift
               away
                 v
Dr:     to the reception---and the girls will send it off-


                        x---------x                        x___
                        ^         ^
        leg & posture       reorientates
            shift              towards
                                  Dr
```

Within the doctor's utterance the patient moves his legs and begins to posture-shift forward, movements which are similar to the patient's actions in taking leave at the completion of the doctor's turn. These earlier movements, an initial attempt to begin to break co-presence, occur at the end of the word "reception," precisely at the first transition-relevance place at which the speaker has indicated the possibility of turn completion. However, following a 0.3-second gap the doctor continues to speak, adding a further turn constructional unit. As he continues, the patient abandons his attempt to leave and realigns his body towards the doctor.

In the following fragment, the patient makes a number of attempts to break co-presence before she actually succeeds.

Fragment 6:4 Transcript 1

```
        (20.00)
P:      It's for a week now (.6) it's for a(.)do I come
        back next week?
        (.7)
Dr:     No you come back in two weeks ⌈time
P:                                      ⌊in two weeks right=
Dr:     =if there's any problem in between you could come
        and see us
P:      Right you ⌈are
Dr:                ⌊otherwise we will see you two weeks on
        Friday
        (.3)
P:      Two weeks on Friday
Dr:     Right?
P:      (Yes) thank you very much
Dr:     Right then
P:      Bye
        (.5)
Dr:     Bye(.)if there's any problems you can tell us (.3)
        right?
P:      Yes(.)right(.)thank you
```

In this instance the doctor finishes writing a prescription, and the patient asks a question concerning the arrangements for the next meeting. An arrangement is made which the doctor goes on to qualify with "if there's any . . ."; then, following the patient's reply, the doctor recycles the proposed arrangement. It is repeated by the patient, and following the doctor's "Right?" the patient thanks the doctor and begins to leave. As she walks out of the room and off camera the doctor adds his final remarks.

Fragment 6:4 Transcript 2

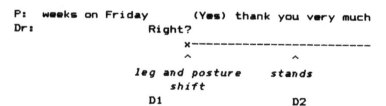

```
P:  weeks on Friday          (Yes) thank you very much
Dr:                  Right?
                        x------------------------
                        ^                    ^
                    leg and posture        stands
                        shift
                        D1                   D2
```

Drawings 1 and 2

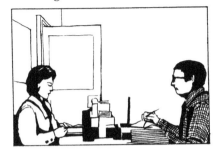 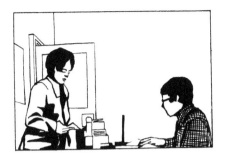

Before successfully taking the doctor's leave the patient makes a number of attempts to begin the process of breaking co-presence. The patient's first attempt occurs towards the end of the doctor's reply to her question. As she utters "in two weeks right" the patient rocks back and forth and readjusts her legs in preparation to stand. Her movements and utterance begin at the end of "weeks," a possible transition place in the doctor's utterance.

<u>**Fragment 6:4 Transcript 3**</u>

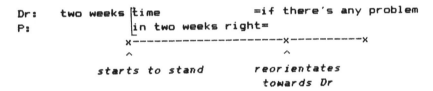

As the patient takes her leave the doctor adds further talk concerning the arrangements; the utterance is latched onto the prior utterance and, given the patient's attempt to leave, is perhaps sensitive to displaying continuation as early as possible. As the doctor continues talk on topic, the patient abandons her leave-taking and reorientates bodily towards the doctor. He qualifies the proposed arrangement, and as he brings the utterance to an end the patient once again attempts to leave as she utters "Right you are."

<u>**Fragment 6:4 Transcript 4**</u>

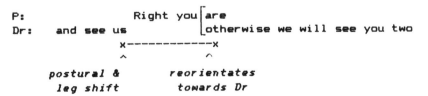

As before, the doctor continues talk on topic – the arrangements for the next meeting – this time actually encroaching upon the patient's own utterance. As he continues, the patient once again abandons her attempt to leave and reorientates towards the doctor. Given these two failed attempts to take the doctor's leave, it is not surprising that at the next possible position she could try to leave ("two weeks on Friday") she remains orientated towards the doctor. This time she awaits "Right?," perhaps a more definite indication that the doctor is going for the end of the consultation.

In Fragment 6:4 therefore the patient makes successive attempts to take the doctor's leave. These attempts are produced as if in second position, as responsive to an utterance by the doctor, rather than being the initial move in a subsequent chain of events. As the patient accepts the proposals to end the business of the consultation she simultaneously begins to take the doctor's leave. As in earlier examples, the patient's nonvocal activity accompanies the acceptance of topic completion of the immediately prior utterance.[5] In accepting topic completion and beginning to quit the surgery the patient finds that the doctor follows her acceptance not with close-relevant components but rather with topic talk. The doctor continues the business at hand, clarifying the arrangements for the next meeting. Almost instantaneously the patient abandons her leave-taking and reorientates towards the speaker, showing involvement in the talk and the other rather than continuing to shift her attention away. Thus the patient monitors the doctor's next move as she begins to quit the surgery, determining whether the other is in fact proposing closure, and is able delicately to tune her nonvocal activity to the very different demands of in- and out-of-topic talk.

Bringing the consultation to an end and taking leave entails the co-operation of doctor and patient. In each instance the doctor produces an utterance, in some cases accompanied by nonvocal actions such as passing objects, that is treated as proposing the end of business – topic completion. In each instance the proposal is accepted by the patient, and except in Fragment 6:4 the doctor takes the consultation's end one step further, initiating the exchange of terminators that lifts the relevance of the turn organization of talk. In Fragment 6:4 the doctor continues topic talk, and in consequence the patient reorientates and cooperates with the speaker's actions. Movement out of the business of the consultation is accomplished through a two-action sequence, through which one party elicits the cooperation of the other in bringing it to an end. In the medical consultation, as in other types of interview, it is the doctor, the interviewer, who typically initiates closure.

Earlier it was suggested that patients coordinated beginning to leave with the turn-by-turn organization of the talk. And in each instance we have found the patient starting to break co-presence at the transition-relevance place of the doctor's prior utterance. Fragment 6:1 reveals in more detail the precision in the coordination between one person's talk and the other's nonvocal activity. The patient monitors the doctor's utterance in the course of its articulation and takes the first opportunity to begin the activity, subsequently abandoning the attempt as the doctor continues. The precise correspondence of the start of the activity and the completion of the utterance unit demonstrates the in-course projectability of the character and structure of the doctor's utterance. It also perhaps reveals the way in which the patient and of course the doctor are preparing for and sensitive to the expected end of the consultation. Management has been sorted out, prescriptions written; these are likely the final moves in the business at hand.

In Fragments 6:1 and 6:4 the patient begins to leave before the actual completion of the business of the consultation and subsequently abandons the attempt and reorientates towards the doctor. Thus in both cases the doctor, actually before topic's end, can infer that the patient is prepared to accept the end of the consultation and duly take his or her leave. In Fragment 6:4 the doctor is aware, as he continues the next utterance, that the patient is prepared to cooperate in closure; in Fragment 6:1, actually within the articulation of the utterance through which he proposes the end of the consultation's business, the doctor receives evidence that the patient is prepared to cooperate and is ready to go. Consequently there may be particular positions within an utterance where the speaker may inspect the visual behaviour of the recipient in order to discern how the utterance will be received following its completion; in the instances discussed here, whether the offer is acceptable.

In each example the nonvocal activity of breaking co-presence occurs within the patient's vocal acceptance of the consultation's end. It also co-occurs with post-topic completion components such as terminal exchanges. Yet the participants avoid engaging in the activity during in-topic or on-business talk. Consequently in Fragment 6:4 we find the patient taking leave and immediately reorientating towards the doctor as further talk concerning the arrangements for the next meeting is uttered. Similarly in Fragment 6:1 the patient ceases leave-taking activities and realigns his body the moment the doctor continues with in-topic talk, even though it is just for the completion of an utterance. The examples throw into relief not simply the coordination between leave-taking and the turn structure of the talk but also the sensitivity to the very different obligations incumbent upon recipients of in-topic as opposed to post-topic talk. As the doctor continues the business of the consultation the patient's responsibilities shift from taking leave to displaying participation in and receipt, through visual behaviour, of the utterance, responsibilities which are lifted following the completion of the business at hand.

Declining to take the doctor's leave

In some cases a proposal to bring the business of the consultation to an end may be declined.

Fragment 6:5 Transcript 1

```
Dr:    I'll get in touch with the hospital and (.7) get
       that report from them
P:     yes
Dr:    but it sounds as if there's nothing to do (.2) at
       the moment you know
P:     yeah
Dr:    O.kay?
       (.5)
P:     so:::
Dr:    You[can start (.3) start on Monday (.3) with that note
P:        [(so)
P:     yeh
       (.4)
Dr:    and err: (.4) that's how was er:: (.)want to know
       it you know(.)want to talk about it you know
```

In this consultation the patient has returned to see the doctor to discuss the results of some tests that the patient had recently undergone at a local hospital. The results have not arrived, and in consequence there is little for the doctor and patient to discuss, save to issue a prescription and a note to return to work. After completing this paper work the doctor produces the utterances beginning "I'll get in touch" and "but it sounds" and within their course passes the note and the prescription to the patient. Given the character of the utterances and the passing of the objects, it seems reasonable to suggest that they serve to propose topic completion and the end of the business for the present time.

On the completion of "but it sounds . . ." the patient could quite properly thank the doctor and begin to take his leave. In fact he utters "yeah" and remains unmoved, orientated towards the doctor. The doctor follows with "O.kay?" – a second attempt to elicit the patient's cooperation in bringing the business of the consultation to an end. In response, following a slight delay, the patient utters "So:::" and simultaneously turns his body towards the doctor. The patient's "So:::" coupled with the accompanying nonvocal action serves to display that the patient is declining to cooperate in ending the business at hand or take the doctor's leave.

Though withholding cooperation in topic closure, the patient's "So:::" passes the floor back to the doctor without progressing the matters in hand. The doctor tries once more. He clarifies the note he has passed to the patient and in doing so proposes the end to the business at hand. Sadly for the doctor, the patient's initial response, "yeh," does not suggest cooperation in bringing things to an end, and following a brief gap the patient continues by elaborating on why he has come. With the patient's "yeh," his third refusal to leave, the patient produces a gesture, a stop sign rather like a policeman holding up the traffic.

Fragment 6:5   Drawings 1 and 2

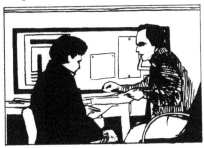 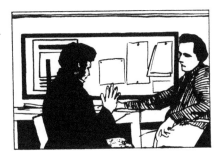

D1   D2
P: So:::...............P: yeh

In Fragment 6:5 therefore we find the patient withholding cooperation in bringing the consultation and its business to completion. In declining to accept the proposal to close, the patient fails to provide the doctor with the necessary resources to allow the interaction to proceed to an exchange of terminators and breaking co-presence. Yet prior to the patient gaining the opportunity to elaborate his reason for the call, the doctor makes successive attempts to close the business at hand, each attempt following the failure of a prior one. Moreover, in declining the proposed close, the patient does not immediately explain why; rather the declination is produced in a mitigated form ("yeh" and "So:::"), keeping the business open rather than opening up a discussion. It is only following the third declination that the patient takes the opportunity to progress the business at hand.

Quite clearly, declining a proposal to finish the business at hand involves rather different actions from acceptance. In the same position as an acceptance, following the proposal's completion, one finds "yeh" and

"So:::" rather than the characteristic "thanks very much." Moreover, far from the patient beginning to leave, we find that bodily orientation remains unchanged or is increasingly aligned with the co-participant's. From simply viewing the patient's orientation alone following a proposal to close, one can gain an inkling of which way the interaction is going. And in some cases it would seem fair to suggest that the speaker's accompanying visual activity allows the party who proposes the close to discern how his utterance is being treated. Components such as "yeh" are occasionally used to accept an offer to end the business at hand, and whether they are treated as acceptances or declinations may depend upon the accompanying visual activity. Vocal and visual co-occur to accomplish a particular action.

In the corpus of data of medical consultations and other forms of professional–client interaction there are very few instances in which a proposal to finish the business at hand is declined; in fact in the data only three instances can be found. On statistical grounds alone one is led to consider that the participants orientate to an acceptance of a proposal to end the business at hand as a "preferred" course of action.[6] By this no personal or psychological preference is implied but rather an orientation to institutionalized sets of options and opportunities where the production of dispreferred actions evidences an array of characteristics that delay, qualify, or account for the action. A preference for acceptance in receipt of proposals to complete the business at hand would be compatible with the organization of related action types such as offers and requests. In Fragment 6:5 we find that the patient's declinations are delayed and done in mitigated form; not immediately raising issues or matters to be discussed, they keep the business open but take it no further. Moreover, in continuing, the patient accounts for his declining to cooperate in bringing the consultation to an end. The doctor on the other hand makes successive attempts to secure the patient's cooperation and only following the declination of the third try temporarily abandons bringing the consultation to an end.

In the rare cases where a proposal to end the business of the consultation is declined, subsequent talk focuses on the earlier problem or related matters. There are no examples in the data corpus of the third possibility occurring, the introduction of a new topic, a different complaint, or whatever. In the light of the literature on the general-practice consultation (for example Balint 1957; Browne and Freeling 1976; Byrne and Long 1976) and data gathered in interviews with practitioners, this is quite surprising, for one of the frequently voiced nightmares of general practice is the patient who as the consultation draws to an end or even on leaving the surgery introduces a new problem. It is referred to as the "by the way" syndrome,[7] and tradition has it that it is at moments like these that patients introduce the "real" problem, not infrequently the underlying psychosocial reasons for their illnesses.

One reason for the relative absence of the introduction of previously unmentioned topics in the closing section of the consultation, either in response to a proposal of topic completion or "misplaced" elsewhere, might be related to the fact that the consultations were being video recorded. More likely perhaps, it appears that if patients are suffering from more than one complaint, they frequently announce their multiple problems at the beginning of the consultation in response to the topic-initiating utterance. If new topics, however, are produced unannounced, then they typically emerge towards the end of the diagnostic phase of the consultation before the doctor prepares the management of the complaint. Consequently on the rare occasions a proposal to finish the business at hand is declined, patients typically seek continuation of prior topics rather than the introduction of a new topic; and if the "by the way" syndrome does occur then it emerges earlier in the medical consultation, often before the details of management are given. The general absence of the introduction of new problems towards the end of the consultation perhaps also bears tribute to the monotopicality of medical encounters, an orientation to a single reason for a visit by both doctor and patient.

Reopening the consultation

As Schegloff and Sacks suggest (1973), closing sections are "porous"; they are open at any point to procedures for reopening topic talk.

Fragment 6:6 Transcript 1

```
        (25.00)
Dr:     O.kay?
P:      O.kay thanks very much Doctor Taloussi
        (.6)
Dr:     Yer can have these tablets if you're not (.2) free
        from pain in a weeks time then come again an
P:                                         yeah
Dr:     see me again
P:      Come back an see ⌈you
Dr:                     ⌊O.kay
P:      Thank you ⌈very much Doctor
Dr:               ⌊bye bye
        (3.0)
P:      Bye bye thankyou
Dr:     Welcome
```

The fragment begins like many others, with the doctor writing a prescription and whilst uttering "O.<u>kay</u>?" passing it to the patient. The patient treats the action as proposing the end of the consultation and accepts with "O.kay thanks . . ." As she speaks she leans forwards and pushes herself out of the chair; by the end of her utterance she is standing and turning away from the doctor. As she begins to walk away, the doctor speaks, continuing talk on topic rather than producing close-relevant components.

The doctor's utterance recommends the tablets for the pain and states that the patient should return if the pain continues. As he begins to speak the patient abandons the course of action in which she is engaged and reorientates towards the doctor. This change in the patient's nonvocal activity begins with the first word of the utterance, "Yer"; by "those," the patient has realigned towards the doctor and is holding her position.

Fragment 6:6   Drawings 1 and 2

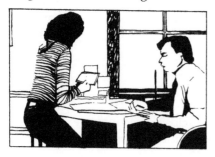 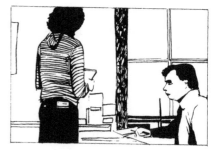

      D1   **D2**
Dr: ------**Yer can have these tablets if you're not**

Thus the reopening of the business of the consultation by the doctor reestablishes certain obligations on the patient, now the potential recipient of an in-topic utterance rather than an interactant collaboratively engaged in closure. The patient abandons her leave-taking and displays recipiency to the speaker. Even by the first word of the doctor's utterance, the patient is able to discriminate the projected utterance as reintroducing a topically relevant item rather than a closing component; "Yer" provides enough for the patient to discern the shift in interactional responsibilities incumbent upon her.

Fragment 6:6 Transcript 2

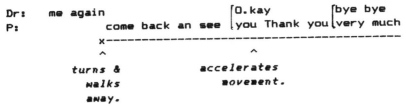

```
Dr:   me again                    ⌈O.kay           ⌈bye bye
P:          come back an see  ⌊you Thank you⌊very much
            x----------------------------------------------
            ^                        ^
         turns &              accelerates
         walks                movement.
         away.
```

The very same utterance with which the doctor reopens the business of the consultation also serves to propose its closure. The patient replies with "come back an see you" and simultaneously reengages her leave-taking. She is standing, and she begins to move away from the doctor slowly and turn her face towards the door of the surgery. These movements are accelerated as the doctor utters "O.kay." It is as if the patient moves slowly until she is certain that the doctor will collaborate in closure. Perhaps also uttering "come back an see you" rather than "thanks" is the patient's way of following the implication of the utterance without committing herself wholeheartedly to closure; vocally and visually she provides the doctor with the opportunity of going either way in next turn.

Examining the behaviour of the patient during the doctor's utterance, one can discern certain movements which occur at the end of "come again." The patient moves her feet and makes a slight turn of the body, movements which appear to suggest the patient is beginning to take leave of the doctor. As with earlier examples, these movements begin at a possible completion point, a transition-relevance place in the doctor's utterance. They start at a position where the if/then format of the utterance could be warrantably finished. The doctor, however, continues, and following the word "pain" the patient abandons the movements, reengaging leave-taking once more at the actual completion of the utterance. Again we can catch a glimpse of the delicacy entailed in starting to take leave and how it is finely tuned to the internal production of a single utterance.

Thus the reopening of a consultation following the acceptance of topic completion and the start of leave-taking entails the coordination and readjustment of vocal and nonvocal actions. Physical leave-taking occurs naturally and freely with post- or out-of-topic talk; yet the reintroduction of the business of the consultation necessitates forms of interactional participation incompatible with leave-taking. An in-topic utterance as opposed to a closing component reintroduces responsibilities for the potential recipient; in particular her displaying, through posture and gaze, attention to the speaker – responsibilities which are not required for post-topic talk. Consequently the business of the consultation may be continued after its accepted completion, but if it is the co-participants are once more subject to the various nonvocal obligations and responsibilities characteristic of in-topic talk.

Modifying and adding an utterance to secure a close

It was mentioned earlier that in certain cases the doctor is able to discern whether a patient is prepared to accept topic closure even before the completion of the proposal to end. In Fragments 6:1 and 6:4 for example the patient begins to leave at relevant junctions within the talk but, on finding the doctor continuing, abandons the activity and reorientates towards the doctor. Consequently the doctor is able to discern that the patient is prepared to accept topic closure and leave at the earliest opportunity. In contrast, the absence of moves to quit the surgery prior to the actual completion of a proposal to end the consultation may lead the doctor to infer that the patient is not prepared to accept the end of the business at hand.

Fragment 6:5 Transcript 2

```
Dr:    you ┌can start (.3) start on Monday (.3) with that
P:         └(so)
Dr:    note
P:     yeh
       (.4)
Dr:    and er:: (.4) thats how was er:: (.) want to know it
       you know what to talk about it you know
       (.6)
P:     because ┌been so:: (.2) you know bein ┌g in the hospital
Dr:            └yes                          │
Dr:    O. Kay                                └fine
P:         ⌈I don't know you know ⌊(    ) in the present state
Dr:        └                      └will you yer (.) you
Dr:    You phone me (.2) in:: (.7) a week or a fortnight
P:     yeah
Dr:    and I'll tell you::: (.3) if I've got the le:tter:
       (.3)
Dr:    I'll phone them and get the letter you see
P:     yeah
Dr:    and ┌then we can talk about it
P:         └so::: then
P:     Right (.) thank you very mu┌ch
Dr:                               └O.kay?
P:     Bye bye::
Dr:    Bye now
```

As can be seen, the doctor is finally successful in bringing the consultation to an end. In fact precisely at the completion of the doctor's utterance "and get the letter you see" the patient begins to take the doctor's leave. He rocks back and readjusts his legs in preparation to stand and pushes himself up. As the doctor utters "and then we . . ." the patient holds his position and reorientates facially towards the speaker. At "about" the patient reengages the activity of leaving, stands, and quits the surgery.

Turning back over the transcript, there appear to be other positions within the talk where the patient might have accepted the end of the consultation and taken his leave. For example the doctor's utterance "you phone me (.2) in:: (.7) a week or a fortnight" might itself be treated by the patient as proposing a satisfactory solution to the problem and possibly the end of the business at hand. More probably this utterance coupled with the one following was treated as a proposal to end the topic and bring the consultation to a close.

Fragment 6:5 Hypothetical Instance

```
Dr:   You phone me (.2) in:: (.7) a week or a fortnight
P:    yeah
Dr:   and I'll tell you::: (.3) if I've got the letter:
P:    Thank you very much ((begins to leave))
```

On listening to the recording, however, it is difficult to hear "and I'll tell you::: (.3) if I've got the le:tter:," coupled with the earlier utterance, as proposing the end of the business at hand. The intonation contour typically found with proposals to complete topic, a sharp rise and fall, is not present. More precisely "and I'll tell you" sounds as if it might be followed by a unit proposing completion. However, when "if I've got the le:tter:" is produced it has no falling intonation. Throughout the utterance the intonation is kept well up and rises towards the end with the sound stretch on the word "let:ter:." The doctor's utterance is articulated so as to suggest he has more to say, and the patient cooperates by not treating the utterance as proposing topic completion.

Turning briefly to the behaviour of the patient during this stretch, there is little evidence to suggest that he is about to take his leave or is even aware that the interview may be drawing towards an end. During the initial utterance "You phone me . . ." the patient gazes at the doctor, and following "fortnight" he remains still, continuing to face the doctor. The patient maintains this orientation, continuing to gaze at the doctor during "and I'll tell you:::" and in the subsequent gap shifts his body slightly towards the co-participant. Hence as the doctor continues with "if I've got . . ." he is faced with a patient who is providing no indication of preparing to leave and certainly giving no visual acknowledgement of the arrangement being proposed. In this light, it is as if the doctor decides within the course of the utterance to abandon the proposal to complete the business at hand and add an additional utterance.

It seems reasonable to suggest that in the course of speaking the doctor infers the possibility of an upcoming declination and alters the activity in which he is engaged. Rather than risk the possibility of a declination and all that it might entail, the doctor articulates the utterance so that it projects more to follow. In this way the doctor avoids having the utterance responded to there and then as a proposal to complete topic talk and provides himself with the opportunity of adding further talk. In continuing, the doctor clarifies the arrangements and firms up the offer to contact the hospital. The additional utterance successfully secures the cooperation of the patient in bringing the consultation to an end. To put it rather differently, the patient, by providing no evidence within the course of the doctor's utterances that he is prepared to take his leave, is withholding cooperation in bringing the consultation to an end. In this way he elicits a more explicit offer from the doctor concerning the results of the tests. Thus in the course of an utterance we find a speaker inspecting the visual activity of a recipient and assessing prospectively how the utterance will be responded to. In consequence he modifies the utterance in which he is engaged and adds further talk so as to secure a particular form of response, an acceptance of the proposed management and thereby cooperation in closure.

Discussion: the disintegration of mutual involvement

Breaking co-presence in the medical consultation is systematically co-ordinated with the turn-by-turn organization of talk. Beginning to take leave co-occurs with an acceptance of a proposal to end the business at hand. The patient positions the nonvocal activity of taking leave to start at the completion of the proposal, and in many instances by the end of the vocal acceptance the patient is standing, ready to quit the surgery. Just as acceptances to candidate topic completions are displayed through the accompanying visual activity, so in declining patients remain orientated towards the doctor and produce a vocalization which keeps the topic open. Proposals to finish the business at hand, immediately following their occurrence, establish an interactional location for their acceptance or declination and particular forms of nonvocal activity. The utterance generates the relevance of a particular vocal and nonvocal activity; patients are obliged to break co-presence if they decide to accept topic completion.

In the course of taking leave the business of the consultation may be reopened. The reintroduction or continuation of talk on topic sets up very different demands on the interactants from terminating the consultation. Speakers reorientate towards their potential recipients, and recipients, engaged in breaking co-presence, abandon the activity and turn facially and posturally towards the speaker. In-topic talk, even a single utterance, reintroduces the relevancies associated with being a recipient, behaviour which is incompatible with the demands of taking leave. Consequently within the domain of the consultation's end we find examples of interactants delicately shifting their forms of participation with respect to the turn organization and topicality of the talk. Whether the utterance is in- or post-topic places very different responsibilities and obligations on the recipient, and recipients finely tune their participation in the course of the utterance to the demands it establishes.

Unlike many of the phenomena discussed elsewhere in these chapters, breaking co-presence is an episode of nonvocal activity. Even so it is found that this large chunk of activity is finely organized with respect to the production of talk. The activity itself assumes a turnlike character, positioned as it is within a slot rendered through a prior vocalization, tuned as it is to transition-relevance places in the developing talk. Moreover this chunk of visual activity is produced with respect to broader features of talk; it is coordinated with utterance and topic organization. Breaking co-presence and taking leave are only appropriate, and then required, following the completion of the business at hand. Yet even though their occurrence is tied to the overall organization of the consultation, it is delicately coordinated with the utterance-by-utterance organization of the talk and the forms of participation required therein.

A relationship between an episode of nonvocal activity and the business of the consultation occurs elsewhere in interaction between the doctor and the patient. Establishing co-presence with the doctor freely occurs with opening talk such as greetings, identity checks, and discussions concerning who the patient is. Yet the business of the consultation rarely begins before the parties have completed the course of action through which they establish co-presence. Of course in many cases movement into the business of the consultation is locally coordinated with the end of the preceding utterance, the finish of reading the records, or a display of recipiency. In others, however, topic initiation is precisely tuned to the patient having brought the activity of establishing co-presence to completion. Thus, as in closings, in the beginning of the consultation we find a relationship between certain utterance types and a body of visual activity.

Bringing the consultation to an end is a progressive, step-by-step process in and through which doctor and patient cooperate and coordinate
their actions. Gaining the co-participant's cooperation in bringing the
business of the consultation to an end allows the doctor to initiate a next
exchange, in many cases a terminal exchange, through which the participants lift the relevance of the turn-taking machinery for talk. Accompanying the participants' movement out of the business of the consultation and a state of incipient talk is physical leave-taking and dismantling
the face-to-face orientation characteristic of much of the medical interview. In bringing the consultation to an end the participants progressively
step out of a common focus of involvement, and though at any moment
within the course of closing doctor and patient are free to reintroduce
talk on topic and the physical alignment it entails, there comes a time
when this is no longer possible; they are out of each other's reach.

In stepping from a state of mutual involvement the doctor and patient
become less aware of and are seen to be less aware of each other's actions
and activities. With their movement out of talk they realign the focus of
their attention and take on tasks seemingly unrelated to the actions and
activities of the other. Of particular significance in the realignment of
involvement, in its disintegration, is the shift in the visual orientation
of the interactants and the point at which they can no longer monitor
the details of each other's nonvocal behaviour.

Fragment 6:1   Transcript 4

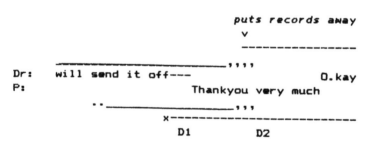

Recall that the patient accepts the proposal to bring the business of the
consultation to an end and begins to take his leave. As the patient accepts
topic completion and takes his leave, the doctor turns away from the
patient. In turning away from his cointeractant the doctor does not simply
turn to one side as he might during the course of an utterance; rather
he swings his head down towards the floor and begins an activity –
removing the patient's medical records from the desk and placing them
on the floor – not unlike the way one begins to clear up as a guest leaves.

The moment the doctor begins to turn away, the patient follows, shifting his gaze directly away as he quits the surgery. Just as the doctor waits until he finds the patient accepting the proposal and taking leave before turning away, so the patient turns away only following the doctor's shift elsewhere. Finding the patient leaving warrants the doctor's action; finding the doctor turning away confirms the patient's decision to leave and warrants his turning away. Each move warrants the former and provides grounds for the next.

Fragment 6:1   Drawings 1 and 2

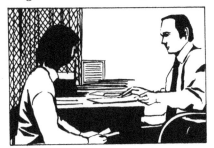 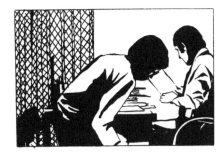

Thus, by the production of the first part of the terminal exchange, the doctor and patient are no longer visually orientated towards each other. Both doctor and patient are involved elsewhere, engaged in activities not sequentially relevant to the other, and certainly not requiring each other's participation. As talk is brought to a close doctor and patient are no longer attending to or monitoring each other's actions, nor are they obliged to be; rather it is incumbent upon each participant to disattend to the action of the other. Visually orientating towards the other person might well elicit some response and raise the possibility that, in realigning attention to the other, the doctor or patient was attempting to initiate an activity and perhaps reintroduce some topically coherent, previously unmentioned matter.[8]

Within the consultation interactants require the attention of others in order to accomplish particular actions and activities. In encouraging others to participate in a certain fashion, a person establishes the interactional and sequential significance of the actions and activities in which he or she is engaged. Here at the consultation's end the doctor and patient mutually realign the focus of their attention and their forms of participation. As they break co-presence and bring talk to completion, the doctor and patient synchronize their actions so that they focus on specific and unrelated spheres of involvement; they accomplish a state where they disattend to the actions of the other even though they may still be in each other's presence. This is not to suggest that the participants may not be sensitive to the actions and concerns of the other, prepared to reestablish mutual involvement at a moment's notice, but rather that they display a civil inattention and appear involved in an activity at hand until the moment at which they are no longer able to monitor each other's behaviour or reopen the consultation.

7. Postcript: the use of medical records and computers during the consultation

One has reached the conclusion that the key to good general
practice is the keeping of good clinical records. Time and again
one has seen a quick glance through a well-kept record card
provide either the diagnosis or an essential point in treatment.
Taylor 1954, p. 35

We believe that a compatible computer system could (and
should) be in widespread use in general practice in five years,
and adopted by virtually all practices in ten years.
Royal College of General Practitioners 1980, p. 42

As Weber pointed out in his classic theory of bureaucracy, files and documents are an essential feature of the modern organization, both in the public sector and the advanced institutions of capitalism. The modern medical organization is no exception. Both time and money are devoted to documenting information concerning the transactions between personnel and their clients. An example of such documents is the medical record card. As even the most cursory visit to a medical organization reveals, a great deal of energy is directed to recording and retrieving from documents the medical biography of patients. Taylor's remarks quoted at the beginning of this chapter reflect a widespread concern in primary care with the importance of medical record cards to good clinical practice.

Medical record cards in general practice consist in large part of brief descriptions of consultations, each consultation warranting a description, a single entry in the records. Though brief, the descriptions typically contain details concerning the assessment and management of a case and whether any referrals, sick notes, and prescriptions were given to the patient. Though the entries appear rough and crude, at least to a lay observer, practitioners regularly use the medical record cards to serve a whole variety of purposes. For example practitioners often design the beginning of a consultation with respect to information gathered from the records, or, when faced with uncertainty concerning the nature of a particular illness, a doctor may turn to the records for hints to or con-

153

firmation of a certain diagnosis. For the general practitioner the records provide a factual version of a patient's medical biography and can be used as a reliable source of relevant information throughout the consultation and other dealings with patients. Thus the importance of the documentary descriptions of consultations lies not just in the fact that they constitute a record, but also in that they are resources in the organization of day-to-day professional conduct. Doctors rely upon the records; they expect them to contain certain sorts of information and to be adequate for their conventional uses. Reading and writing the descriptions found in the records are an integral part of conducting professional activity; the descriptions are necessary for both the assessment and management of illness.

Medical practitioners therefore use the record cards during the consultation with the patient. They frequently need to read and write the records both before the beginning of the consultation and while they converse with the patient. In many cases reading the records cannot be left until the patient has quit the surgery or even disclosed all he has to say; information has to be discerned from the cards as issues and contingencies arise during the course of the consultation. Even writing the notes, which one might imagine could be done after the patient has left the surgery, may have to be conducted during the consultation whilst the doctor can recall the precise details worthy of mention. Consequently a bureaucratic feature of modern medical practice, the documentation and retrieval of information through a system of records and files, is pertinent to the interaction between organizational personnel and their clients.

Reading and writing the records whilst the patient speaks

It might be helpful to reintroduce briefly a couple of fragments discussed earlier.

Fragment 3:6 Transcript 1

```
         ((knocks))
Dr:      Come in
         (1.5)
Dr:      Hello
P:       Hello
         (3.4)
Dr:      Err::(.)how are things Mister (.6) Arma⌈n?
P:                                              ⌊Erm:::(.5)
         all right(.)I just err::(1.0)come to (.7)·have a
         look you know about err:::(.7) heerrr: (.4) have
         you got any information from hos:pital
Dr:      No::: (.3) I don't think so (.3) urm:::
```

Fragment 4:7 Transcript 1

```
Dr:    yes yes
P:     to get on that bus::(.)or in the car: (.2) its: a
       case of (uh) I can't breathe:: (.3) hum:::(.) you
       know (.)um::(.) an I'm all: trembly: an::⌈(      )
Dr:                                           ⌊are you
       allright when you get out of the bus or⌈car
P:                                             ⌊sweatin
Dr:    or is it?                               ⌊
       (1.2)
P:     it lasts until I get where I'm going
```

As pointed out earlier, the patient's reply in Fragment 3:6 is fraught with difficulty, including pauses, "erm's "err's," and sound stretches. In reviewing the example medical practitioners have frequently attributed the speech difficulties to the ethnic background of the patient and the possibility that he may not be able to speak English properly. Yet in the first part of the utterance and later in the consultation there are stretches where the patient has little difficulty in talking. For example "have a look you know about" is a reasonable stretch of English providing little evidence of linguistic difficulty. It coincides with the patient receiving the doctor's gaze; as the doctor turns back to the records the patient again runs into difficulties.

The second example is rather different. It will be recalled that the patient, in the course of an utterance, illustrates her difficulties through a series of gestures. They pass unnoticed by the doctor, and she tries once again. For the second time the illustration is ignored, and the patient subsequently attempts to describe vocally the difficulties she has been suffering. Even though the description was initially requested by the doctor, both its visual and vocal components are unacknowledged either during or after their production.

Like many other examples discussed in the preceding chapters, Fragments 3:6 and 4:7 capture a speaker, and in particular the patient, running into difficulties in the production of an activity. These difficulties are systematically related to the behaviour of the potential recipient. In these and other cases the patient is not simply faced with a potential recipient who is looking away but with one who is rather visibly engaged in an activity–reading or writing the medical record cards. As suggested earlier, finding the doctor engaged in the medical records may well lead the patient to conclude that his recipient's attention is at best divided and at worst elsewhere. Gestural activity and speech hesitation may help solve the problems the patient is facing by encouraging the doctor to realign his gaze.

Very briefly, the following capture some of the difficulties which emerge whilst the patient attempts to speak and the doctor reads or writes the medical records. An asterisk marks where the doctor begins to use the records, an "x" where he turns back to the patient.

Fragment 7:1

```
Dr:   Have you got any problems that's worrying you
                                     *
P:    none at all(.)its just that (2.5.) I feel (.2) as
      though I'm breaking up
      (5.0)
      x
Dr:   where do you work
```

Fragment 7:2

```
        *
P:    And me < nerves have been very bad<°me fingers are
      breaking out in rashes and it's really::
      (6.3)
              x
Dr:   yes we got a letter
```

Fragment 7:3

```
                                            *
P:    when I'm going to the toilet it is too hard you
                                        x
      know hhh (.5) too (.3) very(. )very fast pain in
      the bowel.
```

Fragment 7:4

```
          *
Dr:   when do you get that
      (.3)
                                         x
P:    if I've been(.)if I do anything (.4) if I'm you
                       *
      know doing anything uh:: (.7) out of the ordinary
      it starts to return
      (.3)
P:    if I've got to hurry or walk up a hill.
```

In the first instance, though the patient initially produces a negative answer to the doctor's question, she goes on to suggest she has more to add. The doctor then looks away and the patient withholds the projected utterance for nearly three seconds. Notice also that, following a lengthy gap, the doctor pays no attention to the patient's disclosure. In the second example the patient accelerates her utterance, fades out, and leaves the utterance incomplete following the doctor's shift to the medical records. In Fragment 7:3 the patient runs into difficulties following the gaze shift to the records and completes the utterance as the doctor returns his gaze. Finally in Fragment 7:4 the patient makes successive restarts, only continuing the utterance as the doctor turns from the records to the speaker. As he returns his gaze to the records the patient once again runs into trouble, only continuing the utterance as the doctor again looks up from the records, and so on. These various forms of difficulty in the articulation of talk by patients, many of which entail the stalling of the activity, appear to be systematically related to the practitioner's use of the medical record cards. In these as in many other instances, as soon as the doctor ceases using the records and realigns his gaze we find the patient producing and progressing the activity with little apparent difficulty.

In the following fragment the patient makes successive attempts to elicit the gaze of the doctor at the beginning of the consultation. It is drawn from the same consultation as Fragment 2:2.

Fragment 7:5 Transcript 1

```
Dr:   What can I do for you?
P:    Ohhh (.2) um:: (.7) um::: last week on our::::fff
      holiday
      (.7)
Dr:   bet your ⌈pardon
P:             ⌊um: at the beginning you know last week..
```

The doctor is reading the medical record cards as the patient begins to respond to the topic-initiating utterance. As in other examples the speaker delays the actual content of the utterance "last . . ." by producing inbreaths, pauses, and "um's." Coupled with the hesitation at the beginning of the utterance is a gesture in which the patient grabs his stomach and produces a facial expression as if in severe pain. Neither the perturbations in speech nor the gestural activity encourage the doctor to look up from the records, and following successive attempts to elicit the gaze of the doctor the patient begins the content of the utterance. As he utters "last . . ." the patient stretches forward and places his elbow on the desk, and this movement succeeds in encouraging the doctor to turn towards the speaker. As the doctor begins to look up, the patient delays the production of the final words by stretching the sound "our::::fff"; the end of the utterance is produced for a seeing recipient.

Fragment 7:5 Drawings 1 and 2

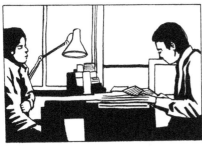 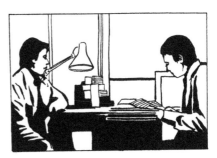

```
          D1                          D2
P:    Ohhh (.2) um:: (.7) um::: last week on our::::fff
```

Faced with a potential recipient who is reading the records, the patient takes the floor to reply and makes concurrent and successive attempts, through speech hesitation and gesture, to elicit the gaze of the doctor prior to producing the content of the utterance. These attempts fail, and the patient begins the substance of the utterance, successfully eliciting the gaze of the doctor during its course. The actual utterance produced by the patient in reply to the doctor's "What can I do for you?" may not, however, be the activity begun at the start. Recall that the patient begins with a gesture and facial expression which embody suffering and in particular severe stomach pain. It might well be expected that this physical illustration of the complaint would accompany its actual description or at least an utterance which elaborated certain details of the suffering. Instead, following a gap and further attempts to elicit recipient participation, the patient produces an utterance which prefaces rather than presents the complaint. The elaborate gesture and facial expression at the start of the reply would appear to bear little relationship to the subsequent utterance. It is as if, on failing to gain the attention of the doctor, the patient withholds the projected activity and instead produces a preface to a description which will be forthcoming following the doctor's reply. In this way the patient takes the floor and replies, whilst not presenting the details of his complaint to a doctor who is inattentive. Alas, the doctor fails to catch the gist of the utterance, whatever it concerns, and the patient has to recycle his prefatory remarks, stalling the consultation still further.

Doctors may not be unaware of the consequences of using the medical records whilst the patient is speaking. In the following example the doctor attempts to read the records and simultaneously display attention to the speaker. The doctor engages in what is akin to tiptoeing.

Fragment 7:6 Transcript 1

```
Dr:    Oh::: so this is what you've come about tonight is
       it
P:     Well really three things
Dr:    uh hu⎡h uh huh
P:        ⎣um:::
P:     those (.2) because=
Dr:    =yes
P:     they haven't stopped⎡I don't tell anyone (.2) you
Dr:              ⎣yes
P:     know(.)I don::'t (1.8) I'm lucky it's happened
       when I'm on my own
```

In reply to the doctor's question the patient mentions that there are three problems. She goes on to elaborate a difficulty mentioned earlier, dizzy spells in open spaces. Having said she does not tell anyone, the patient continues with "you know(.)I dont::'t" – an utterance which projects more to follow, perhaps an elaboration of why she does not discuss the problem. The patient pauses and on continuing to speak begins a new utterance; the projected elaboration is not forthcoming.

Fragment 7:6 Transcript 2

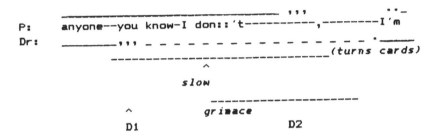

The doctor turns to the medical records and the patient begins to speak almost simultaneously. In fact it might be that the patient begins to speak as she notices the doctor beginning the activity, attempting to draw his attention back to the talk. The doctor, however, remains with the records and following a minigap the patient goes on to propose that she has more to say with "I don::'t." As the patient utters "I don::'t" the doctor slows the activity of turning the pages of the records, lifting the leaf of the page with an exaggerated care as if handling a precious manuscript. At the same time as he alters the pace of the activity the doctor begins to grimace, dropping his chin and tightening his mouth. The doctor's action reminds one of a pupil taking a furtive look at a book during an examination.

Fragment 7:6   Drawings 1 and 2

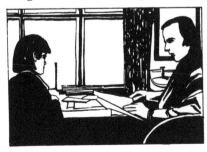 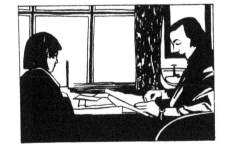

Finding the patient continuing to speak, the doctor behaves as if he is attempting to conduct the activity unnoticed. The way in which he turns the pages of the records has the exaggerated care and slowness of tiptoeing, like stepping forward in the children's game "What's the time, Mr. Wolf?" The accompanying grimace gives expression to the care and delicacy with which the activity is being performed. The articulation of the activity is in almost complete contrast to movements designed to elicit another's gaze. It appears designed to cope with and defuse the potential of a stray movement catching the other's eye; to avoid any slight disruption in the environment of activity. Yet slowing the pace of an activity and beginning to grimace – tiptoeing in the course of using the records – perhaps themselves run the risk of being noticed. If so, it may also be the case that tiptoeing displays a sensitivity to the activity and its production whilst the patient is speaking, showing, if noticed, an appreciation of the patient and thereby a continued attention to her utterances. Whatever, it fails. The patient pauses, continuing to speak only after the doctor looks up from the records.

Thus though a doctor may attempt to avoid the possible consequences of using the medical records whilst another is speaking, his actions may still disturb the activity. In many cases the patient simply withholds an utterance or part of an activity, pausing in its course, until the doctor finishes the activity in which he is engaged. Other devices which allow the speaker to delay the utterance include sound stretches, "um's" and "err's," and the recycling of components of the utterance, devices which delay an utterance and serve to encourage recipient action. In some instances the projected activity, be it an utterance and/or physical display of the complaint, is abandoned altogether with the speaker beginning afresh following the realignment of the recipient's gaze. And given the progressive, utterance-by-utterance development of talk, it is not at all certain that the speaker, having failed to accomplish the activity at one moment, will gain a subsequent opportunity to provide the details in question.

In using the medical records whilst a patient is speaking a doctor may not only undermine the opportunity for the production of activity but miss details and information presented by the patient.[1] There are numerous examples in the data of the doctor failing to catch what the patient is saying whilst reading or writing the records, and requesting its repetition. More significant perhaps, doctors are also found to initiate lines of inquiry on matters covered by the patient earlier in the consultation whilst the practitioner was using the records, where there is no evidence to suggest that the patient's earlier remarks are taken account of. It is almost as if the doctor is able to converse and structure his actions and activities whilst he is using the records, but in so doing misses a range of detail. However, though it is possible to run through the data and find rather gross evidence of doctors apparently missing details said whilst they are engaged in the records, it is of course impossible to say how much other information may be lost by the doctor attempting to divide his attention in this way.[2]

Doctors rely upon patients to provide information concerning their complaints and difficulties; the assessment and management of illness, diagnosis and prognosis, are dependent upon the patient's presentation. In using the medical records whilst the patient is presenting the complaint the doctor may disadvantage both himself and the patient. The patient may run into difficulties in disclosing a complaint and undermine the details and information being provided to the doctor. It may of course be that an activity is delayed, withheld until the recipient realigns his gaze, the consultation becoming a little longer than necessary. However, patients may abandon particular activities or the doctor may miss information provided by the patient. It could be that such information is redundant, yet it is perhaps foolhardy to assume such details are unnecessary. It is better perhaps that the doctor decides when listening to a patient what is relevant or irrelevant rather than curtail both the ability to listen and the patient's actions in such a haphazard fashion.

The use of the medical records in the consultation and more generally the behaviour of the practitioner as a recipient are pertinent to the findings of other studies in the field. The ways in which practitioners use the records can serve to increase or decrease the opportunity available to patients to disclose information; they may encourage or discourage the patient. Take for example Byrne and Long's study (1976) of verbal behaviours in the consultation; the doctor's accompanying visual actions can assist or undermine the opportunities provided through certain types of utterance. The broad-ranging opportunity to disclose information given by an open or reflected question may be severely curtailed if the doctor reads during the patient's reply. On the other hand looking at records whilst asking a closed or direct question may help to delimit the answer further. Thus aspects of the practitioner's visual behaviour provide differential opportunities to the patient to provide information and constrain his behaviour in particular ways.

In producing an activity a patient may not necessarily require the gaze of the recipient; the activity may be articulated with little difficulty even while the recipient reads the medical records. Turning to the records and making notes may even serve to display an appreciation of a stretch of talk. Or for example in disclosing embarrassing information a patient may prefer the doctor to look away. However, reading or writing the medical records rather than simply looking away may render the recipient insensitive to the demands of the speaker. Being involved elsewhere may not just make it more difficult to catch what the patient is saying and doing but render the doctor less able to monitor the immediate requirements of the speaker for his attention. Consequently gestural activity, speech perturbation, and the like, designed to establish a certain orientation from the recipient, may pass unnoticed, and the speaker may have to systematically upgrade his attempts to gain the attention of the recipient. Thus even though patients might not require the gaze of the doctor in the course of an activity, using the medical records rather than simply looking away may render the potential recipient insensitive to the moment-by-moment demands of the speaker and the forms of co-participation he requires.

An additional point: Following a search of the whole corpus of video recordings of the general-practice consultation, it was noted that there is a preponderance of patient-initiated attempts to elicit gaze in consultations where the participants are from different ethnic backgrounds, in particular white British doctors and Asian immigrants.[3] It is also noticeable that many of the more elaborate movements used to attract another's gaze are also found in this type of consultation. A closer look at the data suggests that initial attempts by these patients to elicit the practitioner's gaze pass unnoticed and that in consequence further upgraded attempts are made. It is too early to comment as to why this might be the case; however, one thought is that hesitation in speech by patients from different ethnic backgrounds from the doctor may be treated as difficulties in speaking the language rather than as systematic attempts to elicit the recipient's gaze. Consequently doctors continue to read or write the records, allowing the patient to take his own time, whilst the patient struggles on, making successive and often increasingly elaborate attempts to gain the attention of the potential recipient.

In general practice there is a growing emphasis on the importance of the doctor–patient relationship to the delivery of health care.[4] It is said that a "good" doctor–patient relationship is a prerequisite to the management of the diverse range of complaints, including the psychosocial problems of patients which increasingly confront the general practitioner. It can provide the necessary environment for the discovery of a broad range of relevant information concerning the complaint and provide the conditions for the development of suitable and successful treatment programmes. A relationship, whether doctor–patient or anything else, emerges in and is sustained through the interaction between people, the actions and activities they perform, and the ways in which they receive the sayings and doings of each other. Consequently now the frequent use of medical records in the consultation may not assist the development of a "good" doctor–patient relationship. Besides the aforementioned difficulties, it is unlikely that talking to a doctor who is visibly engaged in reading or writing the records helps the patient establish empathy or contributes to an improvement in the quality of communication.

It is sometimes suggested that the general practitioner has to use the medical records whilst the patient talks to save time. There are of course severe constraints on the time the practitioner has available for each patient; it was reported by the Royal College of General Practitioners in 1973 that the average consultation is less than seven minutes long. This figure conceals of course some variation in the length of consultations, though in the circumstances it might well appear reasonable to reduce contact time with the patient by using the records during the interview. However, besides other difficulties reading or writing the records as a patient speaks may generate, it is found that speakers withhold or delay talk until the recipient's gaze is realigned. It has also been noted that doctors may ask questions concerning matters which were dealt with earlier by patients whilst the doctor was engaged with the records. Consequently using the records whilst the patient is speaking may not necessarily save the time supposed; in fact it may inadvertently lengthen the consultation.

There are ways in which the doctor may use the medical records without running the risk of disrupting the patient's actions and activities or radically increasing the length of the consultation. Take the following couple of examples. The doctor reads or writes the records following the completion of the patient's utterance, allowing the patient to speak uninterrupted.

Fragment 7:7

```
P:    They were poorly at the time and had a temperature
      and he gave them penicillin but they've still got
      a very bad cough
      (.3)
      they've nearly finished the penicillin he gave for
      the two boys
    *(6.0)
Dr:   So×they are well but for the cough?
```

Fragment 7:8

```
P:      And the other cases that I went up for on Friday<
        they put back until my husband's been up to the
        Crown Court
Dr:     so things are better
P:      yeah
Dr:     good that probably makes you feel better than any
        medicine
P:      yes it does
        *(6.0)x
P:      I want to ask you if I can have a pregnancy test
        Doctor
```

In both cases the doctor delays turning to and using the medical records until a second or so following the completion of the patient's utterance, providing the patient with the opportunity to continue if she wishes. In the second example in fact the doctor allows the patient recognizably to complete a particular topic before starting to write the medical records. By delaying reading or writing the records until a second or so following a patient's utterance the doctor can provide an opportunity for talk to be continued, and then if it is not forthcoming collaboratively disengage from the patient to use the records.

If the doctor envisages that he needs more than a brief glance at the records or to jot down a quick note then it may be helpful to tell the patient he is going to use the records. It allows the participants to disengage and temporarily suspend the relevance of the turn-taking organization of talk.

Fragment 7:9

```
P:      And I have been feeling like this for a number of
        years on and off
        (.3)
Dr:     I think I need to look at your records to get
        details of when you saw the doctor last
P:      mmh huh
        *(20.00)
Dr:     Xwhat did...
```

The use of medical records is an essential part of "good general practice" and the delivery of health care in modern industrial society. Medical records are not simply bureaucratic demands on the everyday practice of medical personnel but an integral set of resources which inform the assessment and management of illness. Doctors need to consult the records during the consultation just as it is necessary to document information before it is lost and forgotten. There are ways of using the medical records which avoid the risk of disturbing the activities of the patient whilst preserving the opportunity to read or write the notes throughout the consultation. By positioning the use of the medical records with respect to the completion of particular utterances and activities or announcing the necessity to read or write, the doctor can avoid seeming inattentive as the patient speaks or interrupting an activity in its course. Moreover rendering actual positions where the records are read or written allows the doctor to concentrate on the activity without having to attempt to divide his attention. Rendering positions for using the medical records with respect to turn organization of talk is unlikely to lengthen the consultation or undermine the practitioner's ability to retrieve or document information; it well may assist the flow of communication and even aid the doctor–patient relationship.

Operating computers during the medical interview

In recent years there has been a growing interest in primary health care in the use of computers to assist medical work.[5] The implications of recent developments in microtechnology for the field are enormous, ranging from the computerization of medical record cards to the elicitation of medical histories from patients by computers. In 1980 a working party led by Clifford Kay for the Royal College of General Practitioners suggested that a computer system should be in widespread use by most practices within the 1980s. Though in 1985 it looks unlikely that this deadline will be met, many consider it probable that a system will be introduced into general practice before long.

There are systems which might lead to the demise of the medical consultation itself; for example in a recent study Dare et al. (1977) discuss an experiment with a computer which takes medical histories from patients. However, in the foreseeable future it is more likely that whatever technology is introduced in primary health care will be located in the practitioner's surgery and designed to aid rather than take over consultative practice. It is anticipated that a system will replace the medical record cards and be used for the storage and retrieval of information in patients' medical biographies. But there is also an interest in experimenting with more radical ideas such as computer-assisted diagnosis and programmes designed to aid management decisions. Whatever system is introduced, it is probable that doctors will be using a computer during the medical consultation, and both parties will have to cope with and adapt to the demands intrinsic to the technology. Thus the computer and how it is employed will be relevant to the communication and the relationship between the patient and the doctor.

As far as I am aware there is not an extensive literature concerned with the impact of recent technological developments on social interaction in organization settings. However, along with emergence of Artificial Intelligence and the concern with user-friendly systems, the consequences of using computers are clearly going to be an important issue for the behavioural sciences over the next few decades. The Medical Research Council's Social Psychology Unit at the University of Sheffield has recently been conducting research in this domain, experimenting with a system of computer-aided diagnosis in hospital casualty departments. In 1981 it joined forces with the Department of General Practice at the University of Manchester and conducted a brief experiment with a number of general practitioners. The diagnostic system was placed in a surgery, and the practitioners were asked to conduct a number of consultations using a computer. To avoid harm to actual patients, a number of professional actors highly experienced in playing patients were used to participate in the experiment. The actors played their parts on the basis of sketches of real cases provided by the medical staff. The consultations were then repeated without the presence of the computers in order to draw some comparison. The consultations were video recorded, and a number of social scientists were asked to conduct some preliminary analysis of the data. The following comments are drawn from one of the reports submitted to the departments in question;[6] they are based on the data gathered in general practice and some video recordings of "naturally occurring" casualty consultations making use of computers that the MRC unit was kind enough to make available.

The computer consists of a standard keyboard and a visual display unit (VDU). The system has a limited programme; it is designed to offer a differential diagnosis on the basis of information typed in by the doctor. As the doctor discusses the complaint with the patient, he types the various features of the difficulty such as its symptoms, and the computer provides diagnoses in terms of their probability. In the course of giving information to the system, the computer also recommends further lines of inquiry to the doctor, enabling possible diagnosis to be confirmed or discarded. Thus the computer is used in the prediagnostic and prognostic phases of the consultation, not infrequently whilst the doctor and patient are talking. As one might imagine, using the computer during the consultation has some significant consequences for the interaction between the doctor and patient.

Not unlike use of the medical records, use of the computer by the doctor appears to disrupt the activities of the patient. For example the patient withholds an utterance or pauses within its course until the doctor turns from the VDU to the speaker and abandons the keyboard. Moreover patients perturb their talk whilst the practitioner uses the computer, producing word stretches, "um's" and "err's," recycling earlier components, and restarting utterances. Alongside the speech difficulties we find patients also attempting to attract the doctor's attention through gestural activity and other forms of body movement. And, as with the medical records, we find the speaker emerging from these difficulties once the doctor has abandoned the computer and turned back towards the speaker.

In this way therefore the consequences of using computers whilst the participants are talking are similar to the ways in which the use of medical records can disrupt the activities of another. It is likely that just as speakers may infer that a recipient who is reading or writing may be inattentive to talk, so might a recipient who is typing or retrieving information from a computer. However, unlike the records, the computer is active within the local environment. For example the image on the VDU changes even if the doctor is not using the system, and at times the computer recommends certain lines of inquiry to the doctor. The change of image on the VDU appears to draw the attention of the doctor and undermine his ability to display continued involvement to the patient. In addition the computer's recommendations can serve to initiate a new line of inquiry between doctor and patient and thereby disrupt the natural flow and development of the business of the consultation. Consequently, unlike the medical records, whose use the doctor can postpone or temporarily delay, the computer demands attention at certain points and can interrupt activities in which the participants are engaged.

Talking with computer noise

At times during the consultation the computer emits either a series of clicks or a whirring sound. For intrinsic interest the videotape recordings were investigated to find whether the presence of the noise bore any relation to the communication between the practitioner and the patient. It is found that the doctors do not actually use the computer whilst it produces the noise. The noise occurs when the computer processes information rather than when details are being entered or results delivered. Hence though there appear to be various difficulties in the talk of both participants whilst the computer emits a noise, few of these problems are related to the direct use of the system by the doctor.

To avoid having to wade through a series of lengthy transcripts, a few phenomena which occur in the participants' talk whilst the computer emits its noise will be mentioned. To begin with there are a remarkable number of lengthy silences between the participants' utterances, silences ranging from a few tenths of a second through to several seconds. Unlike many silences one finds in the consultation, they are not occupied by either the doctor or patient engaging in a nonvocal activity such as reading or writing the records or preparing for an examination. A prevalence of pauses in the actual utterances of both the doctor and the patient during episodes of computer noise are also found. Similarly these pauses range from a few tenths of a second to several seconds. As with the silences, there are no accompanying nonvocal activities which explain these continual delays in speech production. In fact, far from shifting their involvement to another activity or concern, the participants remain orientated towards each other and maintain their mutual involvement. These gaps in the talk, both the silences and the pauses, are best characterized as periods of waiting in which the participants retain a state of mutual engagement.

Besides these gaps there are other difficulties in the participants' talk during episodes of computer noise. One of the more striking phenomena in the materials is the frequency of self-repetitions by the speakers. These are instances in which the speaker, either doctor or patient, repeats a word or part of an utterance in the course of a single turn at talk. For example one finds many utterances such as: Dr.: "do, do you drink at all?"; P: "I think that (.) that might help"; or Dr.: "What's going, what's going on with the business at school?" Like silences and pauses, these repeats appear to delay the speaker's production of the utterance; and again close scrutiny of the data reveals no nonvocal actions or activities to explain the vast bulk of these repetitions during episodes of computer noise.

In a recent paper Buckner (1980) reports various findings concerning the nonvocal responses of men and women to background noise whilst they are attempting to speak. Buckner concludes that personality rather than sex differences between speakers explains gestural variation in such cases. With this in mind the data was examined in order to discern any apparent variation in vocal and nonvocal responses to the computer noise by various categories of participant. The sample of course is nothing like valid, but, like Buckner, the inspection found no relationship between the sex of the participant and the vocal and nonvocal activity during the episodes of computer noise. Nor was it found that the doctor and patient were differentially affected by the presence of the noise. However, recurrent types of problems in the participants' talk do emerge that perhaps suggest that in this case response to background noise may not be so much personality-related as something to do with the participant's interactional solutions to the problems at hand.

The computer produces two types of noise, one a repetitive clicking, the other a whirring sound. The two noises are distinct; if the computer is producing one it is not producing the other. The noises occur in episodes; there is a period of clicking noise, followed by a slight pause and then a period of either clicking or whirring. There tend to be more episodes of clicking than whirring. The length of each episode varies, as does the sequence of the episodes. So for example a brief episode of clicking may be followed by a lengthy episode of whirring or a second episode of clicks. Yet when one listens to the episodes some pattern does seem to emerge, if only temporarily.

To examine the relationship between the noise of the computer and the speech of the participants in more detail, an initial attempt was made to transcribe the noise in relation to the speech. The vocal elements of the data were transcribed across the page with accompanying lines to indicate the position of the episodes. A "c" or "w" is marked on the line to show what type of noise the line represents. To assist understanding of the participants' talk and any relation between gaps in speech and the location of episodes, pauses and silences were represented by dashes, each dash being equivalent to 0.1 second. The following is a brief example:

<u>**Fragment 7:10**</u>

```
P:     ..well: I've had---------an then-------------I mean
          c                      c   w                 c   w
       (.)_____(.)__(.)_____(.)____(.)____
P:     I know---------------
       _____(.)_____(.)w___
Dr:    you see it it might affect the treatment
          c
       (.)_____, (silence)
```

The patient's utterance follows a gap of 1.4 seconds in which no speech is articulated but during which the computer is emitting noise. Approximately 0.1 second before the patient utters "well: I've had" there is a pause in the noise of the computer, a gap between episodes. As the computer pauses, the patient begins to speak, and as the patient speaks the computer reengages with an episode of clicking. The patient utters three words, alongside the episode, and then pauses prior to the completion of the utterance. The pause lasts 0.8 second, and the patient attempts to continue her utterance with "an then." During the 0.8-second pause in the patient's utterance the computer disengages and reengages twice. As it pauses for the second time the patient begins to speak, the continuation of the utterance occurring precisely within the brief pause between episodes. And so the process continues. As the computer reengages, the patient ceases her utterance prior to its completion. She only begins to continue in a gap in the noise of the computer. There is then a gap between the patient's utterance and the doctor's which is again filled with the noise of the computer. The doctor begins his utterance in a gap in the noise and then continues with no difficulty after the cessation of the episode of clicking.

In Fragment 7:10, as on other occasions when the participants attempt to speak during the noise of the computer, there appears to be a synchrony between the production of an utterance and the episodic structure of computer noise. It is found that segments of the speaker's utterance and the pauses between the episodes of computer noise are juxtaposed. The speaker coordinates the beginning or segments of the utterance with the pauses in order to begin whilst the computer is silent. As the noise reengages, the speaker stalls prior to the completion of the utterance, only to continue once again in a gap between episodes. Hence one aspect of the delay of speech both at the beginning and within the articulation of an utterance may be related to awaiting a gap in the noise.

The gaps between the episodes are very brief, perhaps 0.2 second. In some instances in which part of an utterance is begun in a gap, there is no discernible break between the completion of the preceding episode and the beginning of the participants' speech. This would suggest that rather than being orientated to the presence of a silence in the noise of the computer, the onset of speech by the participants is positioned with respect to an upcoming completion of an episode. It would seem that the participants may detect when a gap is about to emerge in the noise of the computer and latch the utterance accordingly. This requires the participants to discern a structure in the flow of the episodes and thereby anticipate gaps. The process is analogous to turn taking in talk, inasmuch as utterance positioning by speakers involves an orientation to the projected completion of a turn by a next speaker rather than awaiting a turn's actual completion. What is of course intriguing in this case is that the speaker can infer a pattern in a stretch of computer noise and anticipate the completion of an episode.

The ability of the participants to find a structure in the episodes of computer noise does seem possible when one listens to the data. At

times there is the distinct impression of a pattern or rhythm in the flow
of the episodes. It may remain for several seconds or a few minutes and
then change its structure. But it is perhaps this patterning which provides
the possibility for the doctor and patient to anticipate the completion of
a particular episode. However, given the brevity of the gaps between
the episodes, a speaker will frequently find that as he begins to speak
the computer reengages.

The episodes of whirring emitted by the computer involve stretches
of unbroken noise. The episodes of clicking consist of a series of rapid
clicks differentiated by minute gaps. An attempt was made to transcribe
the periods of clicking in more detail, in particular those in which either
doctor or patient attempted to speak. The transcript of the speech was
laid out across the page and the clicks indicated by the symbol "x." The
arrows indicate the onset position of words. In fact it turned out easier
to position the vocal elements with respect to the internal structure of
the episode than vice versa. The following is a simplified extract from
one of those transcripts.

Fragment 7:11

```
Dr:    ...--I:(.)was fairly sure:(.)that (tablet)....
              v    v      v         v      v
       (.)   xxxxxxxxxxxxxxxxxxxxxxxxxxxxxxxxxxxxxxxx
```

The extract consists of part of an utterance spoken by the doctor and an
episode of clicks. This utterance, like others, begins in the gap between
two episodes; as the doctor speaks the computer reengages. The doctor
produces "I:," pauses, continues with part of his utterance, pauses, and
so on. This utterance, like others that are articulated alongside an episode
of clicking, sounds staggered; not only are there pauses between short
segments of the utterance, but each word, though spoken quickly, is
separated from the next by a slight gap. After repeated listening to the
material, it is found that the words of the utterance each begin in the
slight pause between the individual clicks of the episode. The speaker
appears to coordinate the articulation of speech with the regular, internal
structure of the episode. If this is the case, it perhaps explains the sense
one has on first listening to the data of a rhythm within the episodes of
clicking and the talk of the participants.

It cannot be suggested that the synchrony found in this data between
the participants' speech and the noise of the computer is more precise
or complex than behavioural coordination found elsewhere in human
interaction. It is interesting, however, to note that the participants are

not only coordinating their actions with each other, but simultaneously synchronizing the articulation of these actions with the operations of the computer. The data provides a brief glimpse of the ways in which human social activity is sensitive to the demands of technological environment. A similar point is made by Kendon in consideration of rather different materials:

> There is a small amount of research which suggests that when subjects are exposed to an input that has a rhythmic organization, such as music, they tend to move in time to it . . . and if they are already performing some activity, such as tapping, or typing, they may bring the rhythm of this activity into relation with the rhythm of the input.[7]

As yet it is unknown whether a system of this type will be introduced into medical practice, whether in secondary or primary health care. Even so the data provides a glimpse of the way in which information technology may feature in the communication between the professional and his client. The introduction of certain computer systems into the consultation, for example one that details alternative treatment programmes, should not disrupt communication to any great extent. Such a programme would be generally used following the diagnosis or assessment of the patient's complaint and would therefore not feature in the interview phase of the consultation. Systems for aiding diagnosis or storing details from medical records, however, have to be looked at with far more care, for they will be used as the doctor interviews the patient and will thereby be consequential for doctor–patient communication.

As suggested, in some ways the consequences of using a computer during the consultation, whether it be to aid diagnosis or perhaps to retrieve medical biographies, are not dissimilar to the difficulties that arise from the use of medical record cards. The keyboard and VDU provide an alternative field of attention for the practitioner which he inevitably has to consult during the course of the interview. Using the computer can lead to the patient searching for the attention of the candidate recipient, employing various devices to encourage the doctor to realign his gaze and display recipiency to the speaker. So, as with the use of records, we find the activity being stalled, perturbed, and even abandoned as the doctor types in information or reads from the VDU. But, also as with the records, it is relatively straightforward for doctors to avoid these difficulties; they can postpone using the computer until the completion of an activity by the patient or if necessary announce that they need to use the system, in both ways providing a position for the realignment of participants' attention.

Computers may raise additional difficulties in the consultation. Obviously any system introduced into general practice or any other interactional and organizational setting must be silent. In fact it is remarkable that printers and other noisy equipment have unnecessarily been placed in environments in which organizational personnel such as receptionists are dealing with clients. The noise and activity of a system do, however, raise a more important point. Certain programmes, such as computer-aided diagnosis and perhaps some record systems, may serve to attract the doctor's attention and can structure the activities in which he is engaged. Changes in the information displayed on the VDU and of course any noise may elicit the doctor's gaze and attention, not only distracting him but also perhaps disrupting the patient's disclosure. Moreover certain programmes need to be dealt with at points which they locate, and again these demands may serve to undermine the activities of doctor and patient. And with programmes which advocate courses of action the doctor may find himself steering the consultation in ways that disallow the natural development of discussion between the participants.

Clearly recent developments in information technology have a very important part to play in the delivery of health care, including the medical consultation itself. Even a relatively crude system for the storage and retrieval of the medical biographies of patients could well have immense practical and even economic advantages over the bits of paper and the indecipherable scribblings found in the medical records. Whatever computer system is found the most useful and financially viable in general practice, it seems likely that doctors will continue to communicate face to face with patients in a consultation. In such circumstances it would seem crucial to pilot any schemes and programmes with care before widespread introduction in order to determine how they may affect communication, since it is in the consultation and the partnership of body movement and speech in interaction between doctor and patient that the business of medicine is accomplished.

Notes

1. Video analysis: interactional coordination in movement and speech

1. L. J. Henderson was of course a medical practitioner by training, though the paper published in the *New England Journal of Medicine* is explicitly a piece of sociological analysis. Henderson worked very closely with Parsons, and in fact the fieldwork on which Chapter 12 of *The Social System* was based was conducted with Henderson.

2. It is rather sad in fact that the sociology of health and illness has tended to explore in particular the sick role described by Parsons and paid less attention to his description of the expectations and depositions of the practitioner and the general discussion of the interrelationship of the roles of doctor and patient. The chapter is a masterpiece of sociological theorizing and alone provides many insights into the interaction between doctor and patient and the responsibilities and obligations which lie therein.

3. For further details concerning the influence of the thought and work of Everett Hughes on these and other studies, see Becker 1983; Becker et al. 1968; and Heath 1984c.

4. Byrne and Long's study was based on some earlier research by Hays and Larson (1963) concerned with the interaction between nurses and patients. In the United Kingdom, amongst both the profession and social scientists, it was Byrne and Long's study rather than the earlier study which had significant impact. Moreover there was of course much earlier work on recordings of interaction in the interview, such as Ruesch and Bateson 1951, the collaboration in Palo Alto in the 1950s, and of course Scheflen's studies (1963, 1966, 1973).

5. There are a few exceptions, including Frankel 1983; Friedman 1979; Heath 1982, 1984a, and 1984b; and Pietroni 1976. The studies by Friedman and Pietroni are specific attempts to present the relevance of nonverbal behaviour to a medical readership and are largely concerned with the therapeutic and psychological aspects of visual behaviour, unlike Frankel and Heath, which explore its interactional organization through microanalysis of video. Concerned with a rather different type of substantive domain, an interesting recent study by Erickson and Schultz (1982) examines the interaction between educational counsellors and their clients.

6. For an excellent discussion of the development and the details of what has come to be known as the structural approach to interaction, see Kendon 1979, 1982a; see also Duncan and Fiske 1977 and Scherer and Ekman 1982. There are some parallels between the structural approach and recent de-

velopments in sociology, namely ethnomethodology and conversation analysis, but also significant differences that there is not the space here to discuss (cf. C. Goodwin 1979b).

7. A classic early example of the use of film in social anthropology is Bateson and Mead 1942. In fact early technology in cinematography was developed to provide the possibility of studying movement, especially of animals. As Kendon 1982a points out, by 1898 A. C. Haddon made use of film to record peoples in the Torres Strait islands and in 1901 Baldwin Spencer used the film to examine the behaviour of Australian aborigines. Generally, however, film failed to make much impression on sociological analysis. It might be expected that video, being cheaper, easier to use, and less intrusive, could provide the researcher with a more useful facility than film.

8. See Blumer 1969; Hughes 1958, 1971; and the aformentioned ethnographic work concerning interaction in medical settings.

9. See for example Garfinkel 1967, forthcoming; Garfinkel and Sacks 1970; and Goffman 1959, 1967, 1971, 1979, 1981; and for an excellent discussion of ethnomethodology and conversation analysis, Heritage 1984a.

10. Video data collected by the author was recorded originally on a Shibadin 700, more recently on a National N. V. 3030F videotape recorder, and in the last couple of years on Sony SL C7E and SLC9E videocassette recorders. Various cameras were used, the most efficient of which was a Sony SL 4000 that works extremely well under conditions of poor light. In much of the original data the camera was positioned outside the surgery behind a one-way window such that the camera was only faintly visible to the participants (see Fragment 1:1 in this chapter). On occasions where it was necessary to place the camera in the presence of the participants, every effort was made to render it as unobtrusive as possible. Typically the camera was jacked well up and placed in the corner of the room. On starting to record, the researcher left the room and let the camera run on its own. The recorder itself was placed outside the room or area of filming, so that its operation and replacing tapes or cassettes would not interrupt the action. If the researcher had to remain in the room during recording, then every effort was taken to minimize his presence. For example, where possible the researcher avoided looking into the camera whilst directing it at the participants (Chapter 2 throws light on why) and displayed attention to the equipment rather than to the participants. Moreover sudden or unusual movements were avoided so as not to attract the participants' attention (see Chapter 3). For a related discussion concerning problems and strategies in video recording of naturally occurring interaction, see C. Goodwin 1981a, ch. 1.

Various camera angles were experimented with whilst recording, the best position emerging as approximately (in dyadic interactions) a 50- to 60-degree angle to a line drawn between the two participants. In most of the data, to enable the behaviour of both participants to be included, an "open" lens was maintained. Tragically, much potentially rich data is useless because the researcher/practitioner focuses in and records closeups, thereby losing the behaviour of one or more of the participants. Obviously with more-than-two-party interaction it grows successively more difficult to include all participants within the scope of the camera without making the images so small that they are useless for research. This has made video research into large gatherings extremely difficult, and for these reasons alone studies of visual behaviour in classrooms, lecture halls, public gatherings, and the like remain relatively rare. In a recent project on multiparty and dyadic interaction (ESRC HR/8143) we largely reverted to using data that includes no more than about four or five participants, since the quality of material for larger gatherings proved almost useless for analysis. It should be added that split screens, multicamera systems, and the like frequently generate more difficulties than they solve.

11. The same type of action or activity therefore may be accomplished through different forms of physical movement, the movement gaining its character and force through its interactional position as well as its design. Within the articulation of some actions and activities, for example bidding at an auction or responding to a request, it is unlikely that the same physical movement could accomplish the task on each and every occasion. Consequently we can begin to consider aspects of the local design of movement and the ways in which it addresses the local interactional environment in accomplishing particular actions and activities. None of this is to suggest, however, that certain types of action and activity are not regularly accomplished through similar forms of human movement, in the same way as components such as "Hello" regularly accomplish the same kind of speech act, namely greetings.

12. An essential difficulty in the analysis of visual behaviour and its presentation is the characterization of movement. As Garfinkel 1967; Garfinkel and Sacks 1970; and Sacks 1963, 1972a have suggested, any description is potentially infinite, in that it reflexively creates the phenomenon it describes and a characterization is produced with respect to some set of relevancies. The absence of a widely used or accepted transcription system for body movement and the inability to include the actual data, the video recordings, with this book, render the problem of presenting the material more difficult still. In the studies included in this book, I rely upon description in the text, transcripts, and drawings, attempting to show that these are in accord with the participants' relevancies. Tragically, however, without the video recordings the reader has no way of checking these characterizations. I am, however, very happy to present the original data where this is practically and ethically possible.

13. I use the expression nonvocal or visual in preference to nonverbal, since these chapters deal with movement in general and do not subscribe to delimiting talk in terms of the verbal/nonverbal distinction; for a related discussion, see C. Goodwin 1981a.

14. This is one of the few instances in the whole corpus of data where we find explicit reference to the camera by the participants. It was collected initially during a search through the corpus for examples where the camera and recording might be said to influence the interaction and thereby the analysis, a problem which might be considered an important difficulty for this type of research. A number of points are worth mentioning: (i) if we are to make an empirical case for the effects of recording on interaction, then we need to demonstrate an orientation by the participants themselves in the production of their action and activity to some aspect of the recording/equipment, and there is little evidence to suggest that in the data used in these studies a strong case could be made; (ii) there are very few explicit references to equipment or recording in the data; and (iii) whether video recorded or not, the participants have to coordinate their action, making it recognizable to each other; how this is done is conventional and publicly available and unlikely to be altered by the presence of a camera.

15. Pointing and showing, especially their relation to speech, are dealt with in detail in Chapter 4.

16. See C. Goodwin 1979a, 1980, 1981a; Jefferson 1983b; and Chapters 2 and 3 here for further discussions concerning how pauses may generate recipient activity.

17. For a detailed discussion of the local interactional organization of an iconic or illustrative gesture and the ways in which it can serve to elicit the gaze of a recipient, see Chapters 3 and 4.

18. Much of the analysis reported in the chapters here was conducted on a videotape recorder and in particular a National N.V. 3030E with edit and slow-motion facility. The machine was modified so that the sound track remained on in slow motion, allowing the researcher to simultaneously slow both speech and vision. In fact slow motion does not prove, for various reasons, particularly useful, and much of the analysis was done on repeated viewings at normal speed. All analysis is conducted on copies; it was found that, following no more than a day's repeated viewing of a fragment, the image had begun to fade. Recently the analysis has been conducted using a Sony SLC9E videocassette recorder that has excellent slow-motion facility. The different machines, and in general the equipment this type of research is conducted on, do influence the observations one makes and the phenomena examined. For example videotape recorders such as the National N.V. 3030E are excellent for exploring the relationship between movement and speech but not so suitable for examining the relations between movements as videocassette recorders such as the Sony SL C9E. It is worth noting that for the data on physical examinations (Chapter 5) the Sony SL C9E was indispensable. The research is now conducted using both types of equipment, copies of the data being recorded onto both formats.

    One further point should be added. Film clearly has advantages over video in terms of quality, slow-motion facility (see Kendon 1977, 1979; Scheflen 1973), sound–vision analysis, etc.; but video does have some advantages over film – not just its economics and nonintrusiveness but also in terms of frames per second (it operates at 50 cycles in the United Kingdom). Some work on film has been made on a relatively slow film (as few as eight frames per second), and this clearly has implications for the phenomena one is able to observe.

19. One argument against using clock time is that in coordinating their actions persons are not orientating to the hands of the clock but developing and synchronizing an interactional pace and that it is this that an analyst needs to capture (see Condon and Ogston 1966 and more recently Erickson and Schultz 1982 for a related discussion). It is interesting to note, however, that in a recent paper Jefferson (1983b) has observed a standard metric for gaps of one second plus or minus 0.2 in conversational materials.

20. It should be said, however, that no attempt was made to capture the depth of detail tracked in the studies mentioned here, nor was all the data or the complete consultation mapped out in this way – only segments containing particular phenomena of interest. Again it should be stressed that the maps were drawn for the purposes of analysis, to be used in conjunction with the actual data – the video recording.

21. In tracking the direction of the gaze of the participants for this research every care was taken to determine eye movement and its orientation. It was repeatedly found that eye movement and changes in the direction of a person's looking were accompanied by shifts, however slight, in head orientation. As a way of checking this observation, a number of consultations were recorded in which we shot closeups, focusing on a particular participant

to evaluate the correspondence between his or her eye and head behaviour. The correspondence again turned out to be extremely high, and in some fragments of data where it was difficult to determine precisely eye movement we have relied upon shifts in head orientation. These observations appear to fit with evidence generated in other studies concerned with gaze – studies both naturalistic (for example C. Goodwin 1981a) and experimental (such as Von Cranach and Ellgring 1974). In fact at the distance at which the participants in the bulk of the data corpus were interacting, it may well be that head orientation as well as eye direction serves to provide information concerning the focus of another's gaze. As the research developed it became increasingly apparent that the interactants themselves relied upon shifts in head and eye orientation to infer gaze direction, and over and over again we find persons coordinating a range of actions, both visual and vocal, with these packages of eye and head shifts; Chapters 2, 3, 4, 5, and 7 provide examples. Evidence also emerged in the course of research that interactants themselves may differentiate gaze from eye behaviour, so that for example in Fragment 4:4 we are able to see the way in which the speaker distinguishes the recipient's shift of gaze from actually looking into his eye. In defining and orientating to gaze it does seem likely that interactants use both head and eye behaviour. Clearly though, this is an issue requiring a great deal of further research and one that may well be clarified by both naturalistic and experimental studies such as the recent work on eye movement and cognition.

22. Since video in the United Kingdom runs at 50 cycles per second, photographs of the monitor have to be taken at a speed less than 0.50 so that bars are not caught. It is found that with a Pentax ME Super and 400 a.s.a. film, the best speed is 0.8 second at aperture 5.6. The recording is held on still frame or pause at the appropriate point, avoiding any frame line, whilst the photograph is taken. Drawings are then made of the photograph and reduced for inclusion in the text. Though in principle I would have preferred to use the actual photographs in the book, certainly as a more "honest" representation of the events, for ethical reasons this would have been impossible. It should also be added that because the drawings are a simplified sketch of the photograph they are a much clearer representation of the phenomena than the originals. Hence there are analytic as well as ethical advantages in using drawings rather than photographs, certainly when trying to provide a reader with a brief impression of the action.

2. The display of recipiency and the beginning of the consultation

1. I am afraid that there is not the space here to review and do justice to the varied and complex literature concerned with the organization of gaze; an excellent discussion of a substantial body of the empirical studies on gaze up until the early 1970s can be found in Argyle and Cook 1976, and more recent discussions can be found in Scherer and Ekman 1982 and Beattie 1983. The growing interest in treating gaze in terms of action and activity can be found of course in works of Goffman, for example 1963, 1967, 1971; C. Goodwin 1979a, 1980, 1981a; M. H. Goodwin 1980b; and Kendon 1967, 1977.

2. There is in fact a slight flicker of the lids midway in the gap. It appears to be responsive to a movement by the doctor as he turns the pages. The patient subsequently keeps her eyes closed as before. The way in which movement can attract another's gaze is discussed in the following chapter. For the purpose at hand it is interesting to note how the patient, even with her eyes

closed, is able to monitor the doctor and is sensitive to shifts in the production of an activity.

3. It is relevant to inquire why the patient produces the posture and gaze shift. In the data there does not appear to be any specific action by the doctor to which the patient's gaze and postural reorientation is immediately responsive. There is, however, a slight head movement by the doctor immediately preceding the patient's action, and one wonders whether the patient may treat this head movement as suggesting that the doctor is about to cease reading the records. In fact the doctor continues to read.

4. The actual beginning is the outcome of a negotiation between the doctor and the patient. The patient puts pressure on the doctor, and the doctor responds but delays the initiating utterance. It is likely that the doctor foreshortens his reading of the records and thereby perhaps initiates the business as he does in order to encourage the patient to recap and disclose information which could be found in the medical records. Sadly for the doctor, the solution does not prove too successful; the patient is not particularly forthcoming.

5. A feature of the organization of the turn-taking organization of talk is that it provides for the possibility of lapses where a recipient does not begin to speak and prior speaker does not continue, the floor becoming neither party's specific responsibility (cf. Sacks, Schegloff, and Jefferson 1974). A display of recipiency is one way in which one party can encourage another to talk and reestablish a common focus of involvement and engagement. See C. Goodwin 1981a, ch. 3, for a detailed analysis of disengagement and reengagement in conversational interaction.

6. It is worth noting that the silence is one second long before the patient produces "⁰tch." Jefferson (1983c) has recently shown that there appears to be a standard metric for silence within conversation of one second plus or minus (0.2). It is interesting to note that the vocal shrug occurs precisely one second into the silence.

7. The patient presents "depression" as her complaint to the doctor. Sitting with her eyes closed may not only avoid pressurizing the doctor into beginning but also contribute to the presentation of her difficulties. There is an old adage that the doctor can tell what's wrong with the patient as soon as he or she walks into the surgery. If the doctor had looked at this patient, it might well have proved correct.

8. Within reason; clearly, the doctor having summoned the patient to the surgery for the consultation, there is a limit to how long she might reasonably expect to await his pleasure before she grows restless. The very fact of having another in co-presence, coupled with the environment of expectation movement into the business at hand, constrains the doctor's opportunity to read the medical record cards. Yet one thing is on his side: The activity is being done for the patient rather than for his own indulgence.

9. See Chapter 3 for details concerning the way in which movement is used to elicit gaze. It also addresses in detail how successive attempts to elicit gaze may be modified or upgraded in order to achieve an action, given earlier failures.

10. For a recent discussion concerning bodily focused activity, self-preens, and the like from a rather different perspective, see for example Bull 1981, 1983. It is interesting to find that whatever other concerns such actions satisfy, in face-to-face encounters they are interactionally coordinated. For instance, as mentioned here, they may occur in juxtaposition to a shift of gaze by another. It also appears that they occur in juxtaposition to a cointeractant's bodily

focused activity, a sort of reciprocity of movements, not unlike those described in Scheflen 1973. In Fragment 2:9 we find an example of an interactant perhaps inadvertently picking his nose in response to another's actions, revealing perhaps the way in which we can all, for some interactional reason, find ourselves engaging in quite untoward activities.

11. The display of recipiency therefore appears to perform two tasks simultaneously: responding to a prior action and eliciting a next. In this way the sequential structure of the sequence pause–gaze has qualities not unlike the summons–return sequence described by Schegloff (1968, 1972) and the characteristic nonterminality of such sequence types. The return to a summons itself constrains the other to produce an action or activity, the grounds for the summons in the first place. In this way a summons–return sequence may serve as prefatory to a subsequent activity, itself constraining the doer of the first to produce the activity. For further details of how gaze figures in such prefatory work, see Chapters 3 and 4 and C. Goodwin 1981a, ch. 2.

12. Owing to lack of space I have omitted some instances here which are almost akin to "side sequences" in talk (cf. Jefferson 1972). They are instances in which a recipient, in the course of another's talk, becomes temporarily involved in an unrelated activity; the utterance is withheld as the activity begins and is continued or restarted on its completion. In many cases the recipient's shift of gaze away and its realignment mark the beginning and end of the activity for the speaker and provide the focus for coordinating his utterance.

13. In multiparty consultations which involve a young child and a parent(s), especially when it is the child who is ill, doctors frequently address some remark to the child and attempt to encourage the child, if of an age, to speak. This exercise typically occurs after the various exchanges in the opening sequence and prior to the (successful) initiation of topic, in the position where one would expect to find the topic-initiating utterance. It is difficult and unimportant in this case to say whether "O.kay: Rob" is a serious attempt to begin the consultation or not; whatever, the co-participants go to a great deal of trouble to encourage Rob to speak. Strong, in his study of paediatric clinics (1979), discusses in detail this sort of preliminary work in which doctors engage with children at the beginning of the consultation.

14. The lip lick is a bodily focused activity, interactionally coordinated, and on this occasion a solution to abandoning talk on finding the potential recipient selecting another speaker. The lip lick displays to the doctor that she is abandoning her attempt to speak.

15. Studies in conversation analysis have examined sequences of talk which preface and project particular activities, for example story prefaces, preclosings, preexaminations, preannouncements, cf. Atkinson and Drew 1979; Sacks n.d.; Schegloff and Sacks 1973; Terasaki 1976; and for an overview Heritage 1984a, b and Levinson 1983. The packages discussed here have some of the flavour of presequences in talk, yet unlike such sequence types they do not project the character of the activity they precede but only that an activity by a particular party is sequentially appropriate if the first move is accepted.

3. Maintaining involvement in the consultation

1. The issue of social integration has remained central to sociological inquiry throughout its development. Clearly the idea of integration used here is very different from more traditional versions, yet detailed analysis of social interaction might and should throw light on the individual's integration in

interaction and thereby society; see for example Simmel 1950, 1969 and in a very different vein Schegloff, Jefferson, and Sacks 1977.

2. In a variety of settings – on the street, in the office, or just sitting at home – one can observe how body movement, such as a gesture, is used to attract someone's attention. Consider for example the way in which a wave across a crowded street can draw a taxi to the kerb; or recall the way in which you might have attempted to attract a friend's notice in class to borrow a ruler or pencil. In these and a multitude of other examples a person produces a movement which encourages another to turn towards him and thereby initiates an encounter, if only very brief. Attracting the gaze of another through body movement may also occur in the course of social interaction. For example, it is said (BBC Radio 4, 6 February 1981 evening concert) that if a conductor wishes to attract the gaze of a particular musician in the orchestra during a concert, he will produce a thrust of the baton towards the person in question, and that will successfully draw his gaze. Or in a very different situation, auctions, it is found that if a candidate bidder wishes to place a first bid on the floor, he may attract the auctioneer's attention and thereby establish his attempt to bid through a particular form of body movement, often a thrust of the catalogue above his head. Whatever such movements are, whether a wave with the hand held high above the head or the slight flex of a leg below a desk, they can be employed to catch another's eye and thereby establish his attention. Professional observers of social life have also noted how a movement may attract another's gaze. Scheflen for example, in his study of communication in a psychotherapy transaction (1973), remarks that body movement occurring outside the direct line of regard of a cointeractant will trigger an orientating reflex, attracting focal vision to the moving part. In a different vein Kendon (1967) records the importance of catching another's eye prior to the exchange of greeting and movement into an encounter, and Lamb and Watson in their light-hearted treatise on the meanings of body movement (1979) discuss some of the difficulties associated with gaining another's attention.

3. I am not happy with this rather top-heavy way of describing the structure of the movement: "gaze-realignment sequence"; but the phrase is a way of capturing the very tight sequential ordering of the two actions and the inferences its organization can generate. In one sense the sequence appears to have the character of a summons–return sequence described by Schegloff (1968, 1972): "In order to use the term 'sequence' in a strong fashion – to refer not merely to 'subsequent occurrence' in the sense of the successive positions of the hands of a clock, but rather to a specifically sequential organization – a property called 'conditional relevance' was proposed to hold between the parts of the sequence unit. When one utterance (A) is conditionally relevant on another (S), then the occurrence of S provides for the relevance of the utterance A. If A occurs, it occurs (i.e. is produced and heard) as 'responsive to' S, i.e. in a serial or sequenced relation to it; and, if it does not occur, its non-occurrence is an event, i.e. it is not only nonoccurring (as is each member of an indefinitely extendable list of possible occurrences), it is absent, or 'officially' or 'notably' absent. That it is an event can be seen not only from its 'noticeability,' but from its use as legitimate and recognizable grounds for a set of inferences (e.g. about the participant who failed to produce it)" (1972, p. 76). Yet in another sense the sequence is much lighter than a summons–return sequence, where the summons might pass unnoticed and be ignored, and on occasions is designed to allow just this possibility. In Fragment 3:1 we find a rather strong version of the phe-

nomenon; but in others they are far more delicate, and the movement, though retaining sequential relevance and implication, gently encourages another to reorientate. One difficulty of course is that in describing and showing the phenomenon one initially selects the more blatant instances, though they are by no means the most interesting.

4. This is a deliberately crude rendition of the fragments to give an impression of the way in which movement can serve to encourage recipient participation with, rather than within, the utterance. As noted above in Fragment 3:2, an additional couple of words are tagged on following the arrival of the recipient's gaze. In Fragment 3:1 the speaker attempts to secure the gaze of the recipient prior to the content of the utterance and on failing resorts to eliciting gaze alongside the talk.

5. From the data of medical consultations I have formed a collection of examples where in talking about his or her complaint the patient articulates the utterance in such a way as to portray actual suffering at a particular moment. As with this instance, up until that point the patient has given little impression of suffering here and now; it is as if at a certain moment in talking about the complaint he or she begins actually to suffer. It is analogous to the situation where children begin to say why they were unhappy sometime earlier, and begin to cry, as if once again they feel the events as suffered before. It is as if the talk momentarily recreates the feeling. Analysis is being conducted on the organization of this phenomenon as part of our research project concerned with communication in medical settings (ESRC HR/8143).

6. In a recent paper Holmes (1984) also discusses the ways in which a group of recipients are simultaneously but differentially addressed in the same utterance.

7. Jefferson suggests: "In the course of some on-going activity (for example, a game, a discussion), there are occurrences one might feel are not 'part' of that activity but which appear to be in some sense relevant. Such an occurrence constitutes a break in the activity – specifically, a 'break' in contrast to a 'termination'; that is, the on-going activity will resume. This could be described as a side sequence within an on-going sequence" (1972, p. 295). She goes on to exercise in detail the organization of such sequences and their local interactional environments. The intervening sequence in this fragment appears to have a flavour of a side sequence.

8. Medical consultations, like other forms of interaction, are frequented by utterances articulated without the gaze of the recipient. The point is that gestural activity, like hesitation phenomena (cf. C. Goodwin 1979a, 1980, 1981a), can serve to encourage locally a form of participation from the cointeractant(s).

9. There are a number of studies, including Beattie 1978a, b; C. Goodwin 1979a, 1980, 1981a; Kendon 1967, that suggest that the gaze of the speaker, and whether directed to recipient or not, is critical to the organization of the utterance and the demands placed upon a recipient. At every point in the analysis discussed in these chapters I have been keen to determine whether recipient gaze realignments and their local positions in an utterance were regularly coordinated with aspects of the speaker's gaze vis-à-vis the recipient. In an analysis of more than three hundred instance of movement–gaze realignments (see also Chapters 2 and 4), there does not appear to be a recurrent relationship between the location of gaze elicitation and reorientation through body movement and the direction of speaker's gaze vis-à-vis cointeractants. Even in the few examples discussed here it can be seen that in some instances speakers are gazing at recipient during gaze elicitation and in others not; in some instances speakers bring their gaze to the recipient following gaze elicitation and in others not; etc. There are also numerous examples in the overall

collection of a speaker eliciting the gaze of a recipient through movement yet not turning towards the recipient in the course of the utterance. This of course is not to say that speaker's gaze is not pertinent to a range of interactional tasks such as next-speaker selection (see Fragment 3:7) and the like.

10. "As Harvey Sacks has suggested to me in correspondence, our totalitarian fantasy of the harsh knock at the door at three in the morning contains little awareness of the fact that, after all, to use a knock, however harsh, is to acknowledge the territorial rights of the resident" (Goffman 1971, p. 351 n. 57).

11. It is interesting to note that in a recent paper Von Raffler-Engel (1980a) has suggested that children between the middle of their first year and the end of the third year will use dissonance created by interactional dissynchrony as an attention-getting device.

12. The examples drawn from the social-work interview are rather different. In Fragment 3:4 the speaker taps the recipient's leg with her foot, a movement which might be considered questionable. However, it is one of the few instances in which if it were brought into question it might help the interviewer by allowing her to voice her difficulties in dealing with Jennifer. In Fragment 3:7 the sequence which establishes Jennifer as a participant actually lies distinct from the business at hand, entailing a break and return to the main topic. Even so, note that the movement itself does not become the focus of attention.

4. Forms of participation

1. Throughout this and Chapter 3 I use the terms *speaker* and *recipient* for the sake of convenience to designate particular interactants. Both terms stand as a gloss for a variety of ways of participating in interaction. As suggested in Chapter 3 and here in more detail, persons participate in an utterance or activity (even the same utterance; cf. Fragment 3:8) in a host of ways, all of which may display attention to the activity in question. The interest here is in how movement is used to fashion the responsibilities and obligations others have towards the activity. Moreover, as will be seen here, it is not simply that persons speak, but rather that they articulate action and activities in a certain fashion, a form which sets a framework of participation for others within interactional presence. For a related discussion, see Goffman 1981; C. Goodwin 1981a, b, forthcoming; Goodwin and Goodwin 1982, forthcoming. Goffman suggests for example: "The relation of any one such member to this utterance can be called his 'participation status' relative to it, and that of all the persons in the gathering the 'participation framework' for that moment of speech. The same two terms can be employed when the point of reference is shifted from a given particular speaker to something wider: all the activity in the situation itself. The point of all this, of course, is that an utterance does not carve up the world beyond the speaker into precisely two parts, recipients and non-recipients, but rather opens up an array of structurally differentiated possibilities, establishing the participation framework in which the speaker will be guiding his delivery" (1981, p. 137).

2. See C. Goodwin 1981a; Jefferson 1983b; Chapters 2 and 3 above.

3. The "er::m:" not only indicates to the doctor that the patient is beginning to speak and so might require his attention, but also that the patient is taking the floor and as yet withholding the content of the utterance.

4. Fragment 4:4 reveals the ways in which interactants may orientate to whether a person is actually looking at another and if so whether gaze is directed towards the face or eyes, an issue which is central to a distinction between

turning one's gaze towards another and actually looking at the other (see also Chapter 1, note 21). Here we find an interactant rendering gaze towards the face as locally inadequate and encouraging the other to focus on the eye itself. Whether the patient can actually differentiate the doctor's initial focus and the eye inspection from his line of regard, it is impossible to say, but note that the doctor's shift forward provides evidence to infer that he is now looking at the eye. The fragment throws into relief how in eliciting another's gaze we do not typically infer that the other is gazing into our eyes; nor should he be.

5. In one way it is hardly surprising that the doctor's gaze shift to the patient's knee passes unnoticed. The patient is standing looking at her knee, and the doctor is sitting the other side of the desk from the patient. The patient does not directly see the gaze shift but when it is recycled notices a movement on the periphery and coordinates her utterance with it. The environment has a flavour suggesting that almost anything the doctor did, save explicitly decline the story, would trigger the patient.

6. There is an extensive literature concerned with illustrations and iconic gestures and debate as to their differences and function; see for example Birdwhistell 1970; Ekman 1974, 1980; Ekman and Friesen 1969, 1972; Scheflen 1973; and more recently Schegloff 1984. Ekman and Friesen say of illustrators: "But all of these illustrators share the attribute of being intimately interrelated with the concomitant verbal behaviour on a moment-to-moment basis; they are directly tied to content, inflection, loudness, etc. Illustrators can repeat, substitute, contradict or augment the information provided verbally" (1969, p. 77), and Ekman (1974) elaborates different types of illustrative gestures: batons, underliners, ideographs, kinetographs, pictographs, rhythmics, spatials, and deictics. Under those categories, the movements discussed here reveal elements of underliners, ideographs, and kinetographs. Ekman and Friesen also suggest: "Illustrators receive some external feedback from the observer, who will usually pay obvious visual attention, although he may not verbally comment as often on illustrators as on emblems" (1969, p. 77). Like Schegloff (1984), I am unable to find much empirical evidence that illustrators or iconics are directly orientated to visually. Of particular interest in the fragment discussed here is that the speaker is actively attempting to establish the gesture as relevant for visual attention. However, to say that illustrators do not typically require a recipient's gaze specifically at the movement is not to suggest that such movements pass visually unnoticed.

7. Schegloff, Jefferson, and Sacks 1977 reveals in detail the systematics of repair in conversation and discusses the preference for self-correction. C. Goodwin 1981a powerfully demonstrates how self-correction may be used to elicit the gaze of a hearer.

8. This is not to suggest that demonstrative pronouns require a visual inspection of the referent for the determination of their sense; however, in this instance the speaker's accompanying nonvocal action encourages a realignment of visual orientation which encourages attention to the referent.

9. In discussing double-duty utterances Turner is drawing from the analysis of adjacency pairs in utterance organization, for example question–answer, summons–return, greetings; see Sacks 1972b; Schegloff 1968, 1972; Schegloff and Sacks 1973. Though movements–gaze shifts appear to have some properties of summons–return sequences, it would be inappropriate to consider them necessarily organized like other adjacency pairs; see Chapter 3, especially note 3.

10. Transition places in utterance production and turn taking are discussed in detail in Sacks, Schegloff, and Jefferson 1974, and a couple of relevant sections

are quoted in Chapter 6. Unit types of utterance formation such as sentential, clausal, and phrasal provide through their first possible completion, and so on, turn-transition-relevance places where transfer of speakership may occur (see Chapter 6 for further discussion).

11. One explanation for the dominant form of response could be that in many cases the party who elicits the gaze of the other is speaking and that the face represents the productive domain of this activity. Yet at the same moment the person will also be engaged in visual activity which, even when quite elaborate, fails to directly draw the other's eye unless invited; and even in instances when the participants are not speaking and sometimes are beyond each other's vocal range, it is found that gaze goes to the face first and then if necessary elsewhere. Perhaps it is because humans and animals treat the face as the primary source of expression and communication, a convention which is of course central to both inter- and intraspecies interaction; see also Darwin (1872/1934).

12. See Garfinkel 1967 and in particular ch. 3, pp. 77–9. A brief quotation from p. 78 introduces this chapter.

5. The physical examination

1. These essays are collected in Hughes 1958 and 1971, pt. II. For a review of Hughes's work on occupations and work and its relevance to medical sociology, see Heath 1984c. It is worth quoting a further classic statement by Hughes concerning licence and mandate: "An occupation consists, in part, of a successful claim of some people to a license to carry out certain activities which others may not, and to do so in exchange for money, goods or services. Those who have such license will, if they have any sense of self-consciousness and solidarity, also claim a mandate to define what is proper conduct of others toward the matters concerned with their work. The license may be nothing more than permission to carry on certain narrowly technical activities, such as installing electrical equipment, which is thought dangerous to allow laymen to do. It may, however, include the right to live one's life in a style somewhat different from that of most people. The mandate may go no further than successful insistence that other people stand back and give the workers a bit of elbow room while they do their work. It may, as in the case of a modern physician, include a successful claim to supervise and determine the conditions of work of many kinds of people; in this case, nurses, technicians and the many others involved in maintaining the modern medical establishment" (1958, p. 78).

2. Emerson in her excellent paper on the gynaecological examination (1970) depicts some of the competing and contradictory demands, in particular the balance between maintaining the patient as a person yet rendering the body as an object.

3. Many of the examples I discuss here are drawn from different types of examination performed on the chest. The reason is that within the data corpus these are the most frequent types of examination; they are also available on camera, unlike other forms of examination, which require the couch; and they provide very clear examples of the middle-distance orientation.

4. The reasons for the middle-distance look are of course directly tied to issues in Chapter 2 and in particular the elicitive character of gaze and the demands it makes on the recipient.

5. Frankel (1983) notes how a doctor may continue to talk to a child during an examination so as to draw the child's gaze and attention from the field of operation to the speaker's face. The participation obligations entailed as

speaker and hearer in the talk serve to shift the child's orientation to the doctor's face. In his study of paediatric clinics Strong (1979) also discusses related issues.

6. In a number of interesting papers Kendon (1980, 1983; and see also 1982b) has recently explored the structural phases within gestural activity. If we think of movements in their physical articulation as entailing a preparatory phase, an operative phase, and a period of withdrawal then it is found that actions may be performed during any one of these stages, and moreover the actions it performs are not necessarily bound to the apparent physical nature of the movement. In determining the international significance of the movement, its tasks within the context at hand, and the location of these tasks, we can explore not only how it is articulated but also its local consequences.

7. See for example Bloor and Horobin 1975, who discuss the sense in which there is a fundamental conflict underlying the doctor–patient interaction. On the one hand patients are expected to relinquish themselves to the expertise and authority of the medical practitioner and on the other retain expertise in the specific details of their complaints.

8. Consider the following:

```
P:      (_ _ ) feels tender:: ((croaky))
Dr:     yeah
        (.3)
P:      yeah
Dr:     hhh yeah
P:      what is it doctor if you don't think thats a rude
        question (.) is it
Dr:     °hhhhh hh  huh  I  dont  think  a   ru:de
        question<I mean I think its  jus:t::  (.3)
        you know(.)(tt) I think it is:: probably
        pai:n from your hear::tt=
P:      =yeah
```

These assessments are currently undergoing analysis as part of an ESRC-supported research project (HR/8143).

9. For excellent discussion concerning the role and nature of embarrassment in social life, see Goffman 1970 and the fascinating analysis by Ricks of the significance of embarrassment in the poetry of Keats (1974).

6. Taking leave of the doctor

1. There are relatively few studies of the organization of movement and speech within interactional closings. In conversation analysis there are studies by Button (forthcoming), Davidson (1978), Jefferson (1973), and Schegloff and Sacks (1973) dealing with the structures of talk in endings (and movement out of closings) but no work as far as I am aware dealing with nonvocal and vocal action in interactional closings. From a rather different perspective there are studies by for example Firth (1972) and Knapp et al. (1973) which explore movement and speech in partings and farewells but not in the consultation or in terms of the sequential structure of actions and activities.

2. It is reported by doctors that they often feel under pressure to provide treatment to patients even where it is unnecessary. The pressure appears to derive in part from the sequential tie between the disclosure of troubles and offers

of help and management found in professional–client encounters and perhaps in other less formal environments.

3. Parts of this paper draw from aspects of the analysis found in Schegloff and Sacks 1973. For further details, see that paper.

4. Sadly there is not the space in this chapter to deal in any detail with the speaker's nonvocal behaviour during proposals to complete the business at hand. In Fragment 6:1, as in other instances discussed here, we find the speaker producing a postural shift away from the recipient concurrent with and towards the completion of the utterance. Coupled with the character of the utterance, such movements appear to display upcoming topic completion or its proposal. Even so we find that the recipients' movements to break co-presence are recurrently coordinated with the organization of the utterance, not its accompanying visual elements.

5. Instead of saying "thank you very much," as she subsequently does, the patient answers the doctor's earlier utterances with a recycled component of the arrangement, for example "in two weeks right=" rather than the characteristic "thanks" or "thanks very much." It might in fact be that, though the patient begins to take her leave, the doctor treats her utterance as not necessarily closing the business down, perhaps even displaying some slight dissatisfaction with the proposed arrangement. The doctor does propose a next meeting which is one week later than the time mentioned by the patient; in consequence the patient, whose sick note is for one week, will have to return to work before seeing the doctor and perhaps having the note renewed. In continuing, perhaps sensitive to the patient's response, the doctor modifies the arrangement, proposing that the patient can return sooner if she wishes. And finally it is worth noting that with the next meeting and its acceptable timing in the air, the doctor actually following the terminal exchange tags on "if there's any problems . . ."

6. A general discussion of the preference organization of various types of action sequences in talk may be found in Heritage 1984a and Levinson 1983. More specific empirical studies of the preference organization of particular sequences include Atkinson and Drew 1979; Davidson 1984; Pomerantz 1975, 1978, 1984; Schegloff, Jefferson, and Sacks 1977.

7. Byrne and Long (1976) discuss the "by the way" syndrome and meet with more success in finding examples. The ideas concerning the significance of such misplaced items (cf. Schegloff and Sacks 1973) are not unrelated to Balint's pioneering ideas (1957) concerning the nature of the consultation, the collusion of silence, and the ignorance of the psychosocial problem.

8. See Chapters 2 and 3 and the discussion concerning the elicitive character of looking at another.

7. Postscript: the use of medical records and computers during the consultation

1. It has been suggested to me by general practitioners that on occasions looking at the medical records can help the patient disclose delicate information. It is interesting to note that in the classic Freudian position in psychoanalysis therapist and client are unable to see each other and are thereby unable to monitor each other's visual behaviour. Perhaps there is almost a guarantee of attention, though one gathers that therapists are not unknown to fall asleep during the interview, showing perhaps that being able to monitor and so maintain the doctor's visual behaviour may have advantages for both patient and doctor.

2. The best of course that we can do is to run through the data of the consultation

and note in various ways how subsequent inquiries by the doctor fail to display in their design appreciation of earlier remarks, a procedure which of course is thoroughly dependent upon a bunch of assumptions concerning how speakers attend to and design subsequent utterances with respect to earlier tellings. Even stickier of course is attributing these missed bits and pieces to concurrent record use. As for how much information is missed with no explicit evidence, one could never say. With this in mind the issues raised here should be treated at best as no more than some ideas on the significance of record use to doctor–patient communication.

3. It is interesting to note that in their recent study of educational counselling interviews (1982) Erickson and Schultz show that communicational difficulties evidenced through rhythmical distortions in movement tend to occur in interethnic interactions. Given the distribution noted here and given that rhythmical breaks enter into the design of movements used to elicit gaze, the observations in this study appear to tie into those of Erickson and Schultz. These observations also tie into the many issues concerning interethnic interaction examined in detail in the studies by Gumperz and his colleagues (Gumperz 1982a, b; Gumperz, Jupp, and Roberts 1979). Our own research into this area continues as part of ESRC HR/8143 and has been greatly assisted by discussions with John Gumperz, Jenny Cook-Gumperz, Celia Roberts, and other members of the Industrial Language Training Units in the United Kingdom.

4. See for example Balint 1957; Browne and Freeling 1976; Byrne and Long 1976; Pendleton and Hasler 1983.

5. For an overview concerning the impact, uses and potential of computers in primary health care, see Ritchie 1984.

6. I should like to express my gratitude to Professor David Metcalfe of the University of Manchester and Dr. Michael Fitter of the University of Sheffield for providing the opportunity to examine this data. Dr. Fitter was also kind enough, on an earlier occasion, to provide other video data of the use of computers in the consultation.

7. The quotation is found in Merabian 1972, p. 4, and is taken from an unpublished 1967 manuscript by A. Kendon, "Some Observations on Interactional Synchrony," pp. 36–7.

References

Argyle, M. and M. Cook. 1976. *Gaze and Mutual Gaze*. Cambridge: Cambridge University Press.

Atkinson, J. M. 1984. *Our Masters' Voices: The Language and Body Language of Politics*. London: Methuen.

Atkinson, J. M. and P. Drew. 1979. *Order in Court: The Organization of Verbal Interaction in Judicial Settings*. London: Macmillan.

Atkinson, J. M. and J. C. Heritage (eds.). 1984. *The Structures of Social Action: Studies in Conversation Analysis*. Cambridge: Cambridge University Press.

Atkinson, P. and C. C. Heath (eds.). 1981. *Medical Work: Realities and Routines*. Farnborough: Gower.

Austin, G. 1806/1966. *Chironomia; or a treatise on rhetorical delivery: Comprehending many precepts, both ancient and modern, for the proper regulation of the voice, the countenance, and gesture: Together with an investigation of the elements of gesture, and a new method of the notation thereof: Illustrated by many figures*. London 1806. Reprinted, 1966 Carbondale: Southern Illinois University Press.

Austin, J. L. 1962. *How to Do Things with Words*. Oxford: Oxford University Press (Clarendon Press).

Balint, M. 1957. *The Doctor, His Patient and the Illness*. London: Pitman.

Bateson, G. and M. Mead. 1942. *Balinese Character: A Photographic Analysis*. Vol. 2. New York: New York Academy of Sciences.

Beattie, G. W. 1978a. Floor apportionment and gaze in conversational dyads. *British Journal of Social and Clinical Psychology*, 17: 7–16.

1978b. Sequential temporal patterns of speech and gaze in dialogue. *Semiotica*, 23: 29–52.

1979. Planning units in spontaneous speech: some evidence from hesitation in speech and speaker gaze direction in conversation. *Linguistics*, 17: 61–78.

1983. *Talk: An Analysis of Speech and Non-Verbal Behaviour in Conversation*. Milton Keynes: Open University Press.

Becker, H. S. 1983. Everett Cherrington Hughes. *American Sociological Association, Footnotes* (April), p. 8.

Becker, H. S., B. Geer, E. Hughes, and A. L. Strauss. 1961. *Boys in White: Student Culture in Medical School*. Chicago: University of Chicago Press.

Becker, H. S., B. Geer, D. Reisman, and P. S. Weis (eds.). 1968. *Institutions and the Person: Essays Presented to Everett Hughes*. Chicago: Aldine.

Birdwhistell, R. L. 1970. *Kinesics and Context: Essays on Body Motion Communication*. Philadelphia: University of Pennsylvania Press.

Bloor, M. J. and G. W. Horobin. 1975. Conflict and conflict resolution in doctor/patient interactions. In C. Cox and A. Mead (eds.), *A Sociology of Medical Practice*. London: Collier-Macmillan, pp. 271–85.

Blumer, H. 1969. *Symbolic Interaction: Perspective and Method*. Englewood Cliffs, N.J.: Prentice-Hall.

Browne, K. and P. Freeling. 1976. *The Doctor–Patient Relationship*. 2nd ed. London: Churchill Livingston.

Buckner, J. 1980. Seen and not heard: a story of storytelling illustrators. In Von Raffler-Engel 1980b, pp. 275–81.

Bull, P. 1981. *The Social Functions of Speech Related Body Movement*. Final Report for the U.K. Economic and Social Research Council, Project no. HR/6404.
1983. *Body Movement and Interpersonal Communication*. Chichester: John Wyley and Sons.

Button, G. Forthcoming. No close closings. In J. Schenkein (ed.), *Studies in the Organization of Conversation*, vol. 2. New York: Academic Press.

Byrne, P. S. and B. E. L. Long. 1976. *Doctors Talking to Patients: A Study of the Verbal Behaviours of Doctors in the Consultation*. London: H.M.S.O.

Chesterfield, Lord (P. D. Stanhope). 1984. *Letters to His Son and Others*. London: Dent (Everyman's Library).

Condon, W. S. and W. D. Ogston. 1966. Sound film analysis of normal and pathological behaviour patterns. *Journal of Nervous and Mental Disease*, 143: 338–47.
1967. A segmentation of behaviour. *Journal of Psychiatric Research*, 5:221–35.
1971. Speech and body motion synchrony of the speaker and hearer. In D. L. Horton and J. J. Jenkins (eds.), *Perception of Language*. Westerville, Ohio: Merrill, pp. 224–56.

Dare, G. A. W., P. Wigg, J. H. L. Clark, M. Constantinidoce, B. A. Royappa, C. R. Evans, and H. E. de Wardener. 1977. Computers in general practice: the therapeutic effect of taking a patient's history by computer. *Journal of the Royal College of Practitioners*, 27: 477–81.

Darwin, C. 1872. *The Expression of the Emotions in Man and Animals*. London: Murray. References here are to the 1934 London: Watts and Co. edition.

Davidson, J. 1978. An instance of negotiation in a call closing. *Sociology*, 12, no. 1: 123–33.
1984. Subsequent versions of invitations, offers, requests, and proposals dealing with potential or actual rejection. In Atkinson and Heritage 1984, pp. 102–28.

Davis, F. 1960. Uncertainty in medical prognosis, clinical and functional. *American Journal of Sociology*, 66: 41–7.
1963. *Passage through Crisis: Polio Victims and Their Families*. Indianapolis: Bobbs-Merrill.

Donne, J. 1633. To his mistress going to bed. *Elegies*. London. Reference here is to the 1950 Harmondsworth: Penguin Books selection, pp. 88–9.

Duncan, S. Jr. and D. W. Fiske. 1977. *Face to Face Interaction: Research, Methods and Theory*. Hillsdale, N.J.: Erlbaum.

Ekman, P. 1974. Movements with precise meanings. *Journal of Communication*, 26: 14–22.
1980. Three classes of nonverbal behaviour. In Von Raffler-Engel 1980b, pp. 89–103.

Ekman, P. and W. V. Friesen. 1969. The repertoire of nonverbal behaviour: categories, origins, usage and coding. *Semiotica*, 1: 49–98.
1972. Hand movements. *Journal of Communication*, 22: 353–74.
1978. *Manual for Facial Action Coding System*. Palo Alto, Calif.: Consulting Psychologists Press.

Emerson, J. 1970. Behaviour in private places: sustaining definitions of reality in gynaecological examinations. In H. P. Dreitzel (ed.), *Recent Sociology*. New York: Macmillan, pp. 73–100. References here are to the 1973 reprinted version in G. Salaman and K. Thompson (eds.), *People and Organizations*, London: Longman (Open University Press), pp. 358–73.

Erickson, F. and J. Schultz. 1982. *The Councillor as Gatekeeper*. New York: Academic Press.

Esquire Etiquette. 1953. Philadelphia: Lippincott.

Firth, R. W. 1972. Verbal and bodily rituals of greeting and parting. In J. S. La Fontaine (ed.), *Interpretation of Ritual: Essays in Honour of I. A. Richards*. London: Tavistock, pp. 1–38.

Fisher, D. F., R. A. Munty, and J. W. Senders (eds.). 1981. *Eye Movements: Cognitive and Visual Perception*. Hillsdale, N.J.: Erlbaum.

Fisher, S. and A. D. Todd (eds.). 1983. *The Social Organization of Doctor–Patient Communication*. Washington: Center for Applied Linguistics.

Frankel, M. R. 1983. The laying on of hands: aspects of the organization of gaze, touch, and talk in a medical encounter. In Fisher and Todd 1983, pp. 19–55.

Friedman, A. and L. S. Liebelt. 1981. On the time course of pictures with a view towards remembering. In Fisher, Munty, and Senders 1981, pp. 137–55.

Friedman, H. S. 1979. Nonverbal communication between patients and medical practitioners. *Journal of Social Issues*, 35, no. 1: 82–9.

Garfinkel, H. 1967. *Studies in Ethnomethodology*. Englewood Cliffs, N.J.: Prentice-Hall.

Forthcoming. *A Manual for the Study of Naturally Organized Ordinary Activities*. 3 vols. London: Routledge and Kegan Paul.

Garfinkel, H. and H. Sacks. 1970. On formal structures of practical actions. In J. C. McKinney and E. A. Tiryakian (eds.), *Theoretical Sociology*. New York: Appleton-Century-Crofts, pp. 338–66.

Glaser, B. G. and A. L. Strauss. 1965. *Awareness of Dying*. Chicago: Aldine.

Goffman, E. 1959. *The Presentation of Self in Everyday Life*. New York: Doubleday.

1961. *Asylums: Essays on the Social Situation of Mental Patients and Other Inmates*. New York: Doubleday.

1963. *Behavior in Public Places*. New York: Free Press. References here are to the 1966 paperback edition.

1967. *Interactional Ritual*. New York: Doubleday. References here are to the 1972 Harmondsworth: Penguin Books edition.

1971. *Relations in Public*. New York: Basic.

1979. *Strategic Interaction*. Oxford: Blackwell Publisher.

1981. *Forms of Talk*. Oxford: Blackwell Publisher.

Goodwin, C. 1979a. The interactive construction of a sentence in natural conversation. In Psathas 1979, pp. 97–123.

1979b. Review of S. Duncan, Jr. and D. W. Fiske, *Face to Face Interaction: Research, Methods and Theory*. *Language and Society*, 8: 439–44.

1980. Restarts, pauses and the achievement of a state of mutual gaze at turn beginnings. *Sociological Inquiry*, 50, nos. 3–4: 272–302.

1981a. *Conversational Organization: Interaction between a Speaker and Hearer*. London: Academic Press.

1981b. Shifting focus. Paper presented at the 1981 Annual Meeting of the American Sociological Association, Toronto.

1984. Notes on story structure and the organization of participation. In Atkinson and Heritage 1984, pp. 225–47.

Forthcoming. Gesture as a resource for the organization of mutual orientation. *Semiotica*.

Goodwin, C. and M. H. Goodwin. 1982. Participation status: coparticipation in the activity of search for a word. Paper for the International Sociological Association, Tenth World Congress of Sociology, Mexico City.

Goodwin, M. H. 1980. Processes of mutual monitoring implicated in the production of description sequences. *Sociological Inquiry*, 50, nos. 3–4: 303–17.

Goodwin, M. H. and C. Goodwin. Forthcoming. Gesture and co-participation in the activity of searching for a word. *Semiotica*.

Gumperz, J. J. 1982a. *Discourse Strategies*. New York: Cambridge University Press.

Gumperz, J. J. (ed.). 1982b. *Language and Social Identity*. New York: Cambridge University Press.

Gumperz, J. J., T. C. Jupp, and C. Roberts. 1979. *Crosstalk*. London: National Centre for Language Training.

Gurwitsch, A. 1964. *The Field of Consciousness*. Duquesne: Duquesne University Press.

Hall, E. T. 1963. A system for the notation of prexemic behaviour. *American Anthropologist*, 65: 1003–26.

   1966. *The Hidden Dimension*. New York: Doubleday.

   1968. Proxemics. *Current Anthropology*, 9: 83–108.

Hall, K. R. L. and I. Devore. 1965. Baboon social behavior. In I. Devore (ed.), *Primate Behavior: Field Studies of Monkeys and Apes*. New York: Holt, Rinehart and Winston, pp. 53–110.

Hays, J. S. and K. H. Larson. 1963. *Interacting with Patients*. New York: Macmillan.

Heath, C. C. 1981. The opening sequence in doctor–patient interaction. In Atkinson and Heath 1981, pp. 71–91.

   1982. The display of recipiency: an instance of a sequential relationship in speech and body movement. *Semiotica*, 42, nos. 2–4: 147–67.

   1984a. Talk and recipiency: sequential organization in speech and body movement. In Atkinson and Heritage 1984, pp. 247–66.

   1984b. Participation in the medical consultation: the coordination of verbal and nonverbal between doctor and patient. *Sociology of Health and Illness*, 6, no. 3: 311–38.

   1984c. Everett Cherrington Hughes (1897–1983): a note on his approach and influence. *Sociology of Health and Illness*, 6, no. 2: 213–35.

Henderson, L. J. 1935. Physician and patient as a social system. *New England Journal of Medicine*, 212, no. 2: 819–23.

Heritage, J. C. 1984a. *Garfinkel and Ethnomethodology*. Cambridge: Polity Press in association with Blackwell Publisher, Oxford.

   1984b. *Recent Developments in Conversation Analysis*. Warwick Working Papers in Sociology, no. 1. Coventry: Department of Sociology, University of Warwick.

Hinde, R. A. and T. E. Rowell. 1962. Communication by posture and facial expression in the rhesus monkey (Macaca mulatta). *Proceedings of the Zoological Society of London*, 138: 1–21.

Holmes, D. 1984. Explicit–implicit address. *Journal of Pragmatics*, 8: 311–20.

Hughes, E. C. 1958. *Men and Their Work*. Glencoe, Ill.: Free Press.

   1971. *The Sociological Eye: Selected Papers on Institutions and Race (Part I) and Self and the Study of Society (Part II)*. Chicago: Aldine Atterton.

Jefferson, G. 1972. Side sequences. In Sudnow 1972, pp. 294–339.

   1973. A case of precision timing in ordinary conversation: overlapped tag-positioned address terms in closing sequences. *Semiotica*, 9:47–96.

   1974. Error correction as an interactional resource. *Language in Society*, 2: 181–99.

   1978. Sequential aspects of story telling in conversation. In Schenkein 1978, pp. 219–48.

   1979. A technique for inviting laughter and its subsequent acceptance/declination. In Psathas 1979, pp. 79–96.

1980. *The Analysis of Conversation in Which "Troubles" and "Anxieties" Are Expressed*. Final Report for the U.K. Economic and Social Research Council, Project no. HR 4805/2.

1983a. *Two Explorations in the Organization of Overlapping Talk in Conversation*. Tilburg Papers in Language and Literature, no. 28. Tilburg: Department of Language and Literature, Tilburg University.

1983b. *Two Papers on "Transitory Recipientship."* Tilburg Papers in Language and Literature, no. 30. Tilburg: Department of Language and Literature, Tilburg University.

1983c. *Notes on a Possible Metric Which Provides for a "Standard Maximum" Silence of Approximately One Second in Conversation*. Tilburg Papers in Language and Literature, no. 42. Tilburg: Department of Language and Literature, Tilburg University.

Kempton, W. 1980. A rhythmic basis of interactional micro-synchrony. In Key 1980, pp. 67–77.

Kendon, A. 1967. Some functions of gaze-direction in social interaction. *Acta Psychologica*, 26: 22–63. Reprinted in Kendon 1977.

1972. Some relationships between body motion and speech. In A. Seigman and B. Pope (eds.), *Studies in Dyadic Communication*. Elmsford, N.Y.: Pergamon.

1974a. Movement coordination in social interaction: some examples described. In Weitz 1974, pp. 150–68.

1974b. The role of visible behaviour in the organization of social interaction. In Von Cranach and Vine 1974, pp. 29–74.

1977. *Studies in the Behavior of Social Interaction*. Bloomington: Indiana University Press.

1979. Some methodological and theoretical aspects of the use of film in the study of social interaction. In G. P. Finsberg (ed.), *Emerging Strategies in Social Psychological Research*. New York: Wiley.

1980. Gesticulation and speech: two aspects of the process of utterance. In Key 1980, pp. 207–29.

1982a. The organization of behaviour in face-to-face interaction: observation on the development of a methodology. In Scherer and Ekman 1982, pp. 440–92.

1982b. Current issues in the study of gesture. Paper for Seminar on Biological Foundation of Gesture: Motor and Semiotic Aspects, Toronto.

1983. Gesture and speech: how they interact. In J. M. Wremann and R. P. Harrison (eds.), *Nonverbal Communication*. Beverly Hills, Calif.: Sage, pp. 13–45.

Key, M. R. (ed.). 1980. *Nonverbal Communication and Language*. The Hague: Mouton.

Knapp, M. L., R. P. Hart, G. W. Friedrich, and G. W. Shalman. 1973. The rhetoric of goodbye: verbal and nonvocal correlates in human leave-taking. *Speech Monographs*, 40: 182–98.

Laban, R. 1956. *Principles of Dance and Movement Notation*. London: Macdonald and Evans.

Laban, R. and F. C. Lawrence. 1947. *Effort*. London: Macdonald and Evans.

Lamb, W. and E. Watson. 1979. *Body Code: The Meaning of Movement*. London: Routledge and Kegan Paul.

Levinson, S. 1983. *Pragmatics*. Cambridge: Cambridge University Press.

Maurer, D. and T. L. Lewis. 1981. The influence of peripheral stimuli on infants' eye movements. In Fisher, Munty, and Senders 1981, pp. 21–9.

Merabian, A. 1972. *Nonverbal Communication*. Chicago: Aldine.

Montaigne, M. Eyquem de. 1952. *Essays*. Book II, no. 12. Tr. C. Cotton. Chicago: Encyclopaedia Britannica.

Ochs, E. 1979. Transcription as theory. In E. Ochs and F. Schieffelin (eds.), *Developmental Pragmatics*. New York: Academic Press, pp. 43–72.

Parsons, T. 1951. *The Social System*. Glencoe, Ill.: Free Press.

Pendleton, D. and J. Hasler (eds.). 1983. *Doctor–Patient Communication*. London: Academic Press.

Pietroni, P. 1976. NVC in the g.p. surgery. In Tanner 1976, pp. 162–79.

Pomerantz, A. M. 1975. Second Assessments: A Study of Some Features of Agreements/Disagreements. Unpublished Ph.D. dissertation, University of California at Irvine.

  1978. Compliment responses: notes on the co-operation of multiple constraints. In Schenkein 1978, pp. 79–112.

  1984. Agreeing and disagreeing with assessments. In Atkinson and Heritage 1984, pp. 57–101.

Psathas, G. (ed.). 1979. *Everyday Language: Studies in Ethnomethodology*. New York: Irvington.

Ricks, C. 1974. *Keats and Embarrassment*. Oxford: Oxford University Press.

Ritchie, L. D. 1984. *Computers in Primary Care: Practicalities and Prospects*. London: Heinemann.

Roth, J. 1963. *Timetables: Structuring the Passage of Time in Hospital Treatment and Other Careers*. Indianapolis: Bobbs-Merrill.

Royal College of General Practitioners. 1973. *Present State and Future Needs of General Practice*. 3rd ed. Report from General Practice, no. 16. London: Council of the Royal College of General Practitioners.

  1980. *Computers in Primary Care: Report of the Computer Working Party*. Occasional Papers, no. 13. London: R.C.G.P.

Ruesch, J. and G. Bateson. 1951. *Communication: The Social Matrix of Society*. New York: Norton.

Sacks, H. 1963. Sociological description. *Berkeley Journal of Sociology*, 8: 1–11.

  1964–72. Unpublished transcribed lectures. Transcribed and indexed by G. Jefferson. University of California at Irvine.

  1972a. An initial investigation of the usability of conversation data for doing sociology. In Sudnow 1972, pp. 31–74.

  1972b. On the analyzability of stories by children. In J. J. Gumperz and D. Hymes (eds.), *Directions in Sociolinguistics*. New York: Holt, Rinehart and Winston, pp. 325–45. Reprinted in Turner 1974, pp. 216–33.

  N.d. Aspects in the sequential organization of conversation, chs. 1–4. Unpublished manuscript. University of California at Irvine.

Sacks, H., E. A. Schegloff, and G. Jefferson. 1974. A simplest systematics for the organization of turn taking in conversation. *Language*, 50: 696–735. References here are to the reprinted version in Schenkein 1978, pp. 7–57.

Sartre, J. -P. 1956. *Being and Nothingness*. London: Methuen.

Scheflen, A. E. 1963. Communication and regulation in psychotherapy. *Psychiatry*, 26: 126–36.

  1966. Natural history method in psychotherapy: communicational research. In L. A. Gottschalk and A. H. Auerbach (eds.), *Method of Research in Psychotherapy*. New York: Appleton-Century-Crofts.

  1973. *Communicational Structure: Analysis of a Psychotherapy Transaction*. Bloomington: Indiana University Press.

  1974. *How Behavior Means*. New York: Doubleday.

Schegloff, E. A. 1968. Sequencing in conversation openings. *American Anthropologist*, 70: 1075–95.
  1972. Notes on conversational practice: formulating place. In Sudnow 1972, pp. 75–119.
  1979. Identification and recognition in telephone conversation openings. In Psathas 1979, pp. 23–78.
  1980. Preliminaries to preliminaries: "Can I ask you a question?" *Sociological Inquiry*, 50, nos. 3–4: 104–52.
  1984. Iconic gestures: locational gestures and speech production. In Atkinson and Heritage 1984, pp. 266–96.
Schegloff, E. A., G. Jefferson, and H. Sacks. 1977. The preference for self-correction in the organization of repair in conversation. *Language*, 53: 361–82.
Schegloff, E. A. and H. Sacks. 1973. Opening up closings. *Semiotica*, 7: 289–327. References here are to the reprint in Turner 1974, pp. 233–65.
Schenkein, J. (ed.). 1978. *Studies in the Organization of Conversational Interaction*. London: Academic Press.
Scherer, K. R. and P. Ekman (eds.). 1982. *Handbook of Methods in Nonverbal Behaviour Research*. Cambridge: Cambridge University Press.
Searle, J. 1969. *Speech Acts*. Cambridge: Cambridge University Press.
Simmel, G. 1950. *The Sociology of George Simmel*. Ed. K. Wolff. Glencoe, Ill.: Free Press.
  1969. Sociology of the senses: visual interaction. In R. E. Park and E. W. Burgess (eds.), *Introduction to the Science of Sociology*. Chicago: University of Chicago Press, pp. 356–61.
Sociological Inquiry. 1980. Special issue, *Language and Social Interaction*, 50, nos. 3–4.
Sociology. 1980. Special issue, *Language and Practical Reasoning*, 12, no. 1.
Sommer, R. 1959. Studies in personal space. *Sociometry*, 23: 247–60.
Sommer, R. F. and Becker. 1974. Territorial defence and the good neighbour. In Weitz 1974, pp. 252–62.
Stark, L. and S. R. Ellis. 1981. Scanpaths revisited: cognitive models direct active looking. In Fisher, Munty, and Senders 1981, pp. 193–226.
Strauss, A. L., L. Schatzman, R. Bucher, D. Ehrlich, and M. Sabshin. 1964. *Psychiatric Institutions and Ideologies*. London: Collier-Macmillan.
Strong, P. M. 1979. *The Ceremonial Order of the Clinic*. London: Routledge and Kegan Paul.
Sudnow, D. 1967. *Passing On: The Social Organization of Dying*. Englewood Cliffs, N.J.: Prentice-Hall.
Sudnow, D. (ed.). 1972. *Studies in Social Interaction*. New York: Free Press.
Tanner, B. (ed.). 1976. *Language and Communication in General Practice*. London: Hodder and Stoughton.
Taylor, S. 1954. *Good General Practice*. Oxford: Oxford University Press.
Terasaki, A. 1976. *Pre-Announcement Sequences in Conversation*. Social Science Working Papers, no. 99. Irvine: School of Social Sciences, University of California at Irvine.
Turner, R. 1976. Utterance positioning as an interactional resource. *Semiotica*, 17, no. 3: 233–54.
Turner, R. (ed.). 1974. *Ethnomethodology: Selected Readings*. Harmondsworth: Penguin Books.
Von Cranach, M. and J. H. Ellgring. 1974. Problems in the recognition of gaze direction. In Von Cranach and Vine 1974, pp. 415–49.

Von Cranach, M. and I. Vine (eds.). 1974. *Social Communication and Movement: Studies in Man and Chimpanzee.* London: Academic Press.

Von Raffler-Engel, W. 1980a. Development kinesics: the acquisition of conversational nonverbal behaviour. In Von Raffler-Engel 1980b, pp. 133–61.

Von Raffler-Engel, W. (ed.). 1980b. *Aspects of Nonverbal Communication.* Lisse: Swets and Zietlinger B.V.

Wada, J. A. 1961. Modification of cortically induced responses in brain stem of shift of attention in monkeys. *Science,* 133: 40–42.

Weitz, S. (ed.). 1974. *Nonverbal Communication: Readings with Commentary.* London: Oxford University Press.

Index

For EU product safety concerns, contact us at Calle de José Abascal, 56–1°,
28003 Madrid, Spain or eugpsr@cambridge.org.

www.ingramcontent.com/pod-product-compliance
Ingram Content Group UK Ltd.
Pitfield, Milton Keynes, MK11 3LW, UK
UKHW010045140625
459647UK00012BB/1613